The Manual Wheelchair Training Guide

Peter W. Axelson
Jean Minkel
Anita Perr

Editing and Layout by Ben Hubbard & Ted Nagel

Illustrations by Clay Butler

PAX Press

P.O. Box 69
Minden, NV
89423-0069

PAX Press is a division of Beneficial Designs, Inc.

Print - ISBN 978-1-882632-15-2
ePub - ISBN 978-1-882632-16-9
Kindle - ISBN 978-1-882632-17-6

Printed in the United States of America

The Manual Wheelchair Training Guide

Table of Contents

Acknowledgments

This manual was completed with a grant from the Paralyzed Veterans of America's Education & Research Foundations (previously PVA's Spinal Cord Injury Education & Training Foundation). We wish to thank the many people whose assistance and expertise made it possible to develop this training guide.

Manuscript Reviewers and Focus Group Participants

Carole Adler	Santa Clara Valley Medical Center
Brian Arakaki	St. Jude Medical Center
Marty Ball	
Bill Blythe	Beneficial Designs, Inc.
Michael Bush	
Frankie Cassaday	Craig Hospital
Rory Cooper	Human Engineering Research Lab, Pittsburgh
Donald Eastmead	La Bonheur Childrens' Medical Center
Gail Gilinsky	Craig Hospital
Gil Haury	Invacare Corporation
Michael Heckrotte	Curtis PMC
Ben Hubbard	Beneficial Designs, Inc.
Susan Johnson-Taylor	
R. Lee Kirby	Dalhousie University
Kay Koch-Hurst	
Betti Krapfl	University of Colorado
David Kreutz	Shepard Center
LeNae Liebetrau	
Mike Molesky	
Ted Nagel	Nagel Business Graphics
Dorothy Nary	University of Kansas
Mandy Pasternak	
Lupo Quitoriano	Paralyzed Veterans of America University of Southern Mississippi
Ross Rogers	Tennessee Valley Authority
John Schatzlein	American Home Health Inc.
Sharon Vazquez	Beneficial Designs, Inc.
Jamie Skilling	Beneficial Designs, Inc.
Julie Steward	
Kathleen Wong	
Denise Yamada	

Introduction

People who use wheelchairs for mobility and transportation depend heavily on their wheelchair maneuvering skills to accomplish basic living tasks. The variety of environments people encounter present complex skill and safety challenges to wheelchair users and their helpers. Unfortunately, many people are not properly trained in the safe and efficient use of their wheelchairs, which may result in falls and serious injury to wheelchair users and their assistants.

This book was designed to be used by wheelchair users, their families, friends, caregivers, and anyone else who might need comprehensive information about manual wheelchair skills. This manual is also very useful to rehabilitation professionals training wheelchair users in wheelchair mobility skills. The illustrated instructions provide guidance for wheelchair users on how to negotiate indoor environments, obstacles, and outdoor terrain. General hints to prepare for traveling, emergencies, and other situations are also included. In addition, the training guide provides instructions on how to assist someone with a technique and describes the progressions for learning new maneuvers. The principles discussed will help readers learn good riding and assisting habits applicable to any mobility skills they might develop in the future.

The skills and information in this guide will hopefully help increase the independence of wheelchair users, decrease the number of wheelchair accidents caused by the lack of education and training, and limit the frustration caused by those receiving or giving assistance. The wheelchair skills and instructions in this book were compiled with the assistance of expert wheelchair users and rehabilitation professionals. These experienced individuals provided input on the wheelchair techniques, text content, and illustrations.

How to Use This Book

We recommend that new wheelchair users or those who have limited familiarity with them read this guide from cover to cover to learn about all aspects of their use. Those more experienced or familiar with wheelchairs may prefer to skim the table of contents to locate specific topics.

Many of the illustrations contain white and/or black arrows. The white arrows indicate the direction of travel. The black ones indicate the direction the wheelchair user should propel the wheels or handrims.

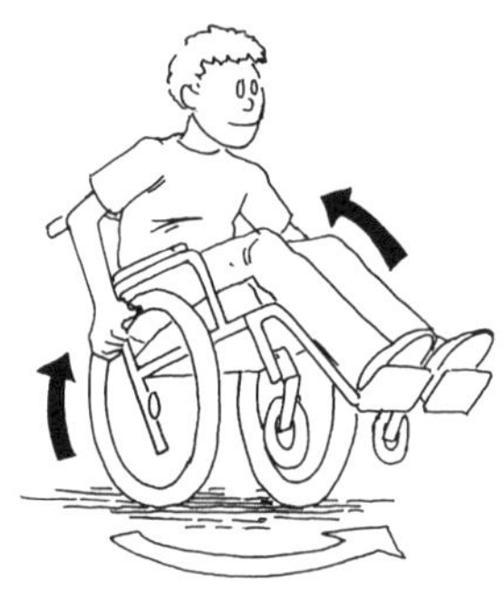

Warnings

This book is based upon work supported by the Paralyzed Veterans of America's Education Foundation and Beneficial Designs, Inc. Any opinions, conclusions or recommendations expressed here are those of the focus group participants and wheelchair experts consulted for the book and do not necessarily reflect the views or policies of the funding organizations or even the authors themselves. Beneficial Designs, Inc. and the Paralyzed Veterans of America do not endorse or recommend any of the specific skills described in this guide and are not responsible for any injuries or deaths that may occur as a result of practicing or performing these techniques.

Wheelchairs are designed to be as small as possible to negotiate indoor environments, and thus may be unstable and require skill to operate outdoors and over uneven terrain. **We have attempted to incorporate all of the manual wheelchair skills that we are aware of into this book, regardless of the potential hazard associated with performing them.** Many of the skills described in this book require considerable skill and/or strength to perform safely. Many of the riskier techniques described here, such as going up and down stairs and escalators, should only be attempted by wheelchair users in emergencies. Performing these techniques incorrectly could result in severe injuries or death if you do not have the requisite wheelchair experience, physical capabilities or assistance. For some people, falling from a wheelchair could result in severe injury or death. If you attempt these maneuvers, enlist the help of a physical/occupational therapist or a therapist/provider who is certified by the Rehabilitation Engineering and Assistive Technology Society of North America (RESNA) as an Assistive Technology Professional (ATP) with a specialty certification as a Seating and Mobility Specialist (SMS) who is experienced in wheelchair training. Use extreme caution while practicing and performing the techniques described in this book. Always enlist very physically capable spotters when attempting more difficult techniques or performing skills for the first time.

Be aware that assisting a wheelchair user as a spotter, helper, or lifter could result in severe injury to you. Obtain training from a RESNA certified Assistive Technology Professional (ATP) with a specialty certification as a Seating and Mobility Specialist (SMS), who is experienced in wheelchair training.

Other Titles from P A X Press:

- The Powered Wheelchair Training Guide
  ISBN 978-1-882632-11-4 Print
  ISBN 978-1-882632-18-3 ePub
  ISBN 978-1-882632-19-0 Kindle
- A Guide to Wheelchair Selection
  ISBN 978-0-929819-06-8 Print
  ISBN 978-1-882632-20-6 ePub
  ISBN 978-1-882632-21-3 Kindle

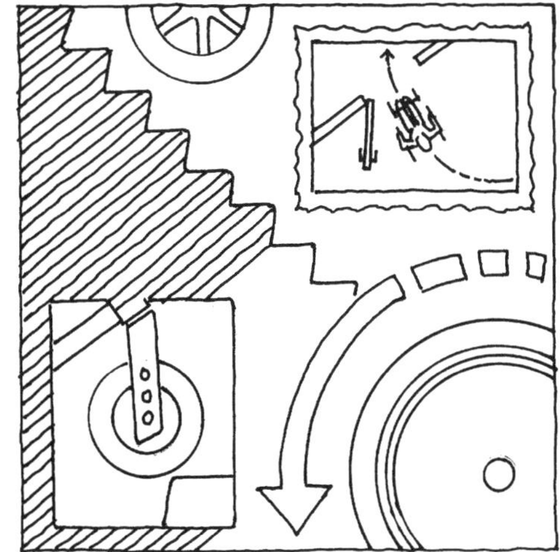

Chapter 1

General Skills

If you are a new wheelchair user, you should get to know your new wheels. While there is no quick and easy method for learning wheelchair skills except practice, Chapter One provides basic information so you can begin using your wheelchair as effectively as possible.

This guide does not cover the many different types of transfers a person should know to be independent in getting around your home, community or when traveling away from your own community. Physical or Occupational Therapists should teach transfers from a wheelchair to bathtubs, toilets, beds, and other areas you might need, like getting in and out of cars. Only floor-to-wheelchair transfers, which are likely to be encountered in emergency situations, are discussed in this guide.

Before practicing the maneuvers in this chapter, read the warning on page vi to learn about the risks involved. Remember that for some wheelchair users, falling may result in severe injury or death.

Sections in This Chapter

Section 1.1

The Owner's Manual

As with all new gadgets, you should read and familiarize yourself with the owner's manual before using your wheelchair. You may be able to find additional information about your wheelchair on the manufacturers' website. Although different wheelchair models may seem similar, each has unique features and adjustments. Many of the secrets to using your wheelchair to its fullest extent lie inside the booklet that came with your wheelchair. You could be injured and/or your wheelchair damaged if it is set up or operated improperly. To prevent this, take a few moments to understand your trusty vehicle before riding off into the sunset.

Read the owner's manual from cover to cover. The information contained in it is very important. Most manuals include information about the following:

- Safety and handling
- Wheelchair parts (list of wheelchair components)
- Accessories and Instructions for Accessories
- Adjustments you can make
- Adjustments your supplier should make
- Maintenance, performance checks, and repair procedures
- Warranty
- Assembly instructions
- Instructions for safe operation
- Instructions for how to inspect for damaged or missing parts
- Common misuse warnings

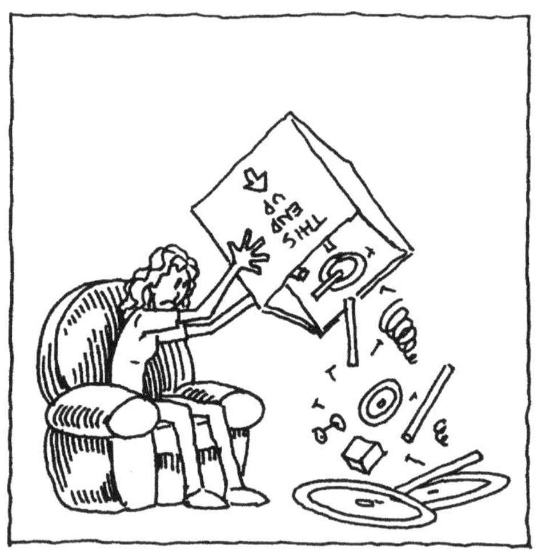

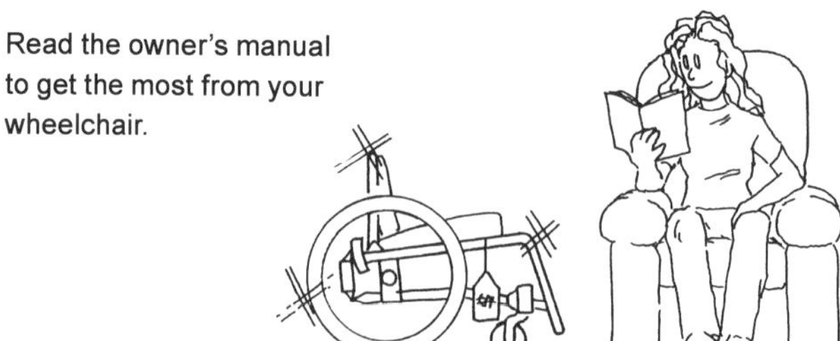

Read the owner's manual to get the most from your wheelchair.

If you have any questions, comments, or concerns about the assembly, adjustment, handling of your wheelchair, or anything in the manual, contact your wheelchair supplier or manufacturer. Do not attempt to adjust components if you do not fully understand the instructions in the manual, as your actions might void the warranty. Do not use your wheelchair until it has been properly assembled and adjusted.

Section 1.2

Set Up and Adjustment

The many hours you will spend in your wheelchair dictate that you should customize it to fit your body. A properly adjusted wheelchair will be more comfortable to sit in, easier to maneuver, and less stressful on your muscles and joints during propulsion. Your wheelchair setup drastically affects your comfort, posture, stability, and ability to use your wheelchair efficiently and effectively.

In a properly adjusted wheelchair, you should be sitting with the best posture that is comfortable for you in order to optimize your function, while preventing pain or deformity. You should have enough room for your knees to fit underneath most table tops. Your foot supports should be high enough off the ground to avoid hitting obstacles in your path. Make sure your wheelchair cushion, back support, and other positioning aids are in place when you make the adjustments to your wheelchair. The position of the rear wheel will dramatically change how hard you are working to push and will impact the long term functioning of your shoulders.

Changes to your wheelchair – One change to your wheelchair will affect the fit of all the other components, so be prepared to spend a fair amount of time on this crucial operation. Ideally, you should enlist the help of an ATP/SMS , certified by the Rehabilitation Engineering and Assistive Technology Society of North America (RESNA), when adjusting your wheelchair.

Wheelchair mobility – Whenever you alter the setup of your wheelchair, check your forward, side-to-side, and rear stability with a spotter to make sure your wheelchair performs the way that you want and that it is not too tipsy. (Section 1.4 Learning Your Limits describes how to experience your limits of stability). After each adjustment, test drive your wheelchair on ramps, different surfaces, and side slopes to make sure your mobility needs have been met.

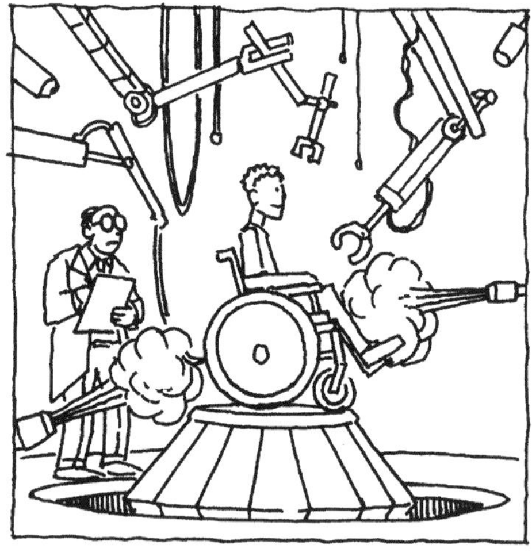

The optimal sitting position for most wheelchair users is with a seat-to-back support angle somewhere between 90-100° and a knee angle in the range of 90-120° of extension. Some wheelchair users like to sit with their feet tucked under their wheelchair creating a tighter knee angle of 70-80°. This may shorten the overall length of your wheelchair and make it easier to maneuver. Shown: 90° seat-to-back support angle and 120° of knee extension.

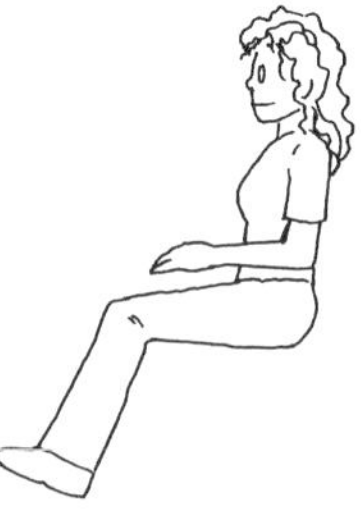

Wheelchair Types

As with automobiles, enterprising inventors have developed many different styles and models of wheelchairs. Each is designed for a different purpose and permits different types of adjustments to be made. There are two basic categories of manual wheelchairs: standard use wheelchairs and rehabilitation wheelchairs.

Standard wheelchair

Standard wheelchairs, also known as depot or institutional wheelchairs, are the no-frills, chromed, steel, or powder coated aluminum workhorses usually found in hospitals, nursing homes, and airports. Standard wheelchairs are designed to be simple to use and durable enough to survive within an institutional setting. The arm supports and foot supports of standard wheelchairs are often welded to the frame and cannot be adjusted or removed. The same standard wheelchair is frequently used by more than one person. Standard wheelchairs are usually sufficient for short-term or infrequent use. They offer the least flexibility in adjustment so they may not be the correct size or configuration for the user. Changes and adjustments must usually be made to standard wheelchairs by replacing components.

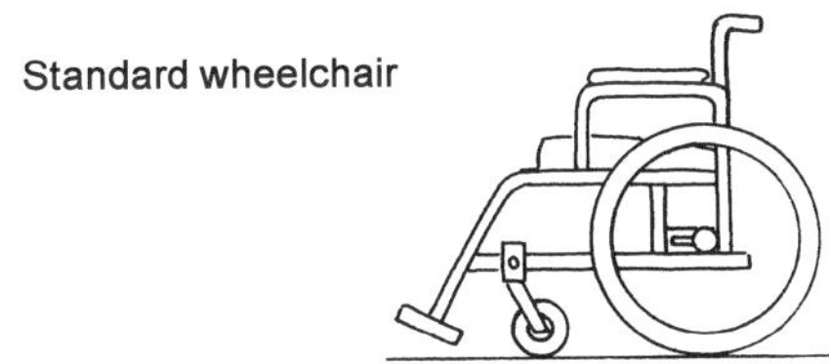

Rehabilitation wheelchairs

Rehab wheelchairs are typically ordered and sized to meet the needs of a specific user. They are generally, but not always, built for a user that depends on the wheelchair full time for mobility. Rehab chairs are generally much more durable than standard wheelchairs so that they will hold up to use in all sorts of indoor and outdoor environments. Rehab chairs are designed and built to be either folding or rigid with a folding back support. The arm supports or skirt guards and leg supports are often adjustable in position and removable to facilitate transfer in and out of the wheelchair. Some rehab wheelchairs have adjustments that can be made to change the back support height or angle, rear wheel fore aft position and height and front caster angle. Most rehab wheelchairs are often lighter in weight to make them easier for the user to get the chair in and out of a vehicle.

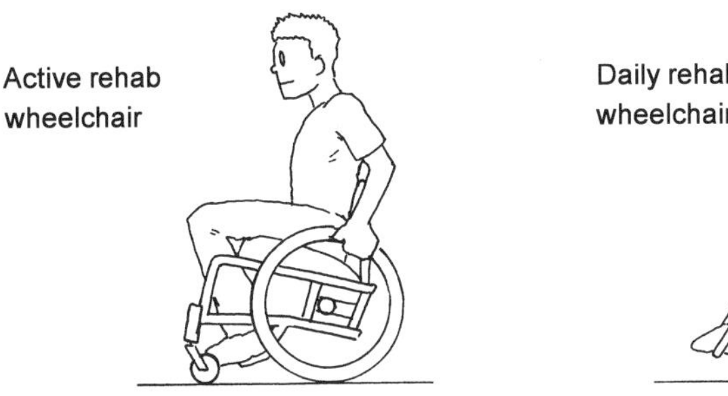

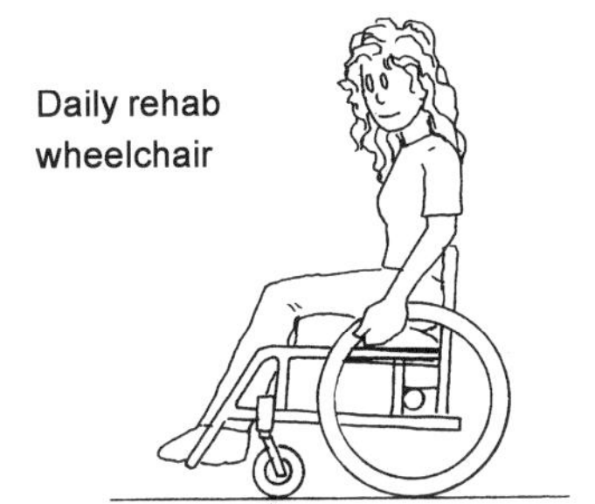

Vertical axle adjustments on Rehab and Standard wheelchairs

Some standard and most rehab wheelchairs offer several vertical adjustment positions for the front and rear wheel axles.

Moving the rear wheel axle up or down will change:

- The seat height
- The seat plane angle
- The back support angle
- The angle of the caster wheels

- The orientation of the frame
- Your ability to reach the handrims

Types of options available on Rehab and Standard type wheelchairs

- Type of back support
- Type of foot support positioning
- Arm support type
- Wheel-lock type and position
- Rear wheel type (e.g. spoke wheels vs. mag (plastic) and size (20", 24", 25", 26" or 27")
- Handrim style, outside diameter, grip diameter, material, shape and method of attachment
- Caster wheel type (e.g. solid versus pneumatic) and size (4", 5", 6" or 8")
- Frame color
- Upholstery color and type

Additional types of adjustments available on Rehab wheelchairs

The most common adjustment that is available on a wheelchair is the fore aft and/or vertical adjustment of the rear axle. This allows the adjustment of the seat height and/or angle which can improve the ability to reach the handrims. Changing the seat angle can also improve the stability and/or function of the user in the chair. Multi-adjustable wheelchairs often have one or more of the following adjustments and/or options available:

- Anti-tippers
- Vertical and horizontal rear wheel position
- Seat support angle and or height
- Front caster position and angle
- Foot support angle, length and or position
- Lower leg support angle
- Back support height and or angle
- Wheel lock position and type
- Seat width and or depth
- Rear wheel camber from vertical to angled out at the bottom
- Arm support height

This training guide describes the proper fitting parameters for each adjustment later in this chapter. Changing or adjusting one part of your wheelchair often changes the position of another part. You will probably have to perform a series of adjustments to achieve the correct fit.

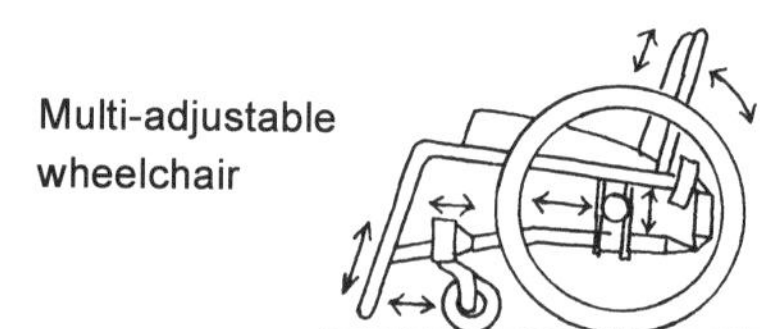

Multi-adjustable wheelchair

Other types of wheelchairs

Add-on power systems

Some add-on power systems require removal of the main drive wheels. Wheels with motors in them are then attached to the chair to amplify the push of the wheelchair user. In this case the handrim is essentially a switch that tells the motors to propel forward when the user pushes on the handrim. The system adds weight to the wheelchair. Batteries must be carried on the wheelchair as well.

Some add-on power systems attach underneath the wheelchair frame and have a separate wheel that touches the ground to power the wheelchair. The Smart Drive™ is a power drive unit that attaches underneath the wheelchair. It senses when the wheelchair user pushes forward on the handrims of the chair and powers the chair to match the strength of the push that the user applies to the handrims. The battery slips under the seat where it hangs on the seat upholstery.

Arm crank wheelchairs

This can be added to a standard manual wheelchair. When the crank drive is attached to the wheelchair it lifts up the front casters of the manual wheelchair. Some wheelchairs are designed for crank driving only.

Basketball wheelchair

These generally have higher seats with very little seat dump, highly cambered main wheels, with a wrap-around frame in the front of the chair to prevent entanglement with other basketball chairs.

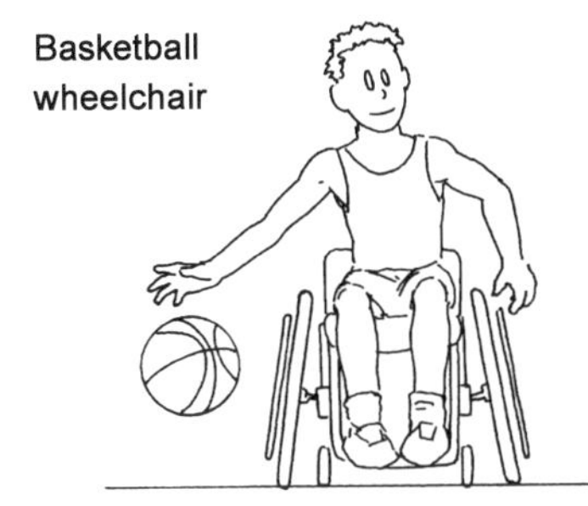

Basketball wheelchair

Beach wheelchair

A wheelchair designed to negotiate sand and soft surfaces. Usually has wider, balloon tires often with large tread and a long wheelbase to provide added stability.

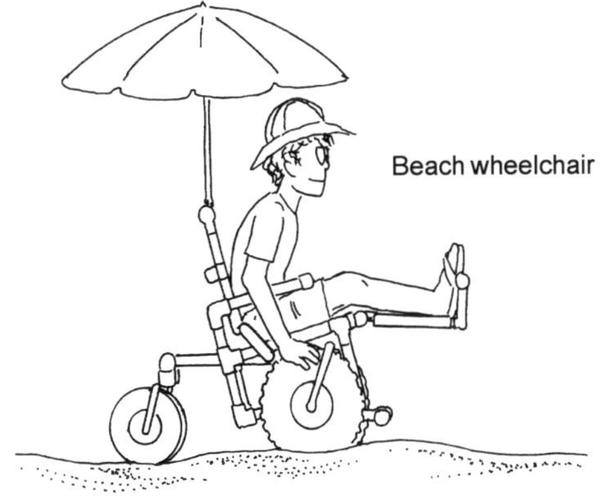

Beach wheelchair

Lever drive wheelchairs

Some lever drive systems can be retro-fitted onto a standard manual wheelchair, others are designed and manufactured for lever drive use only and have no handrims. A lever drive chair can increase the leverage that can be applied to push the wheelchair forward.

Hemi-height wheelchair

Hemi-height refers to a low floor to seat height. Wheelchairs are sometimes set-up with a "lower" seat to floor height to allow a person with hemiplegia to use one hand and one foot for self-propulsion. This style wheelchair is thus often referred to as a "hemi-wheelchair".

Off-road wheelchair

An off-road wheelchair has large knobby tires similar to those on a mountain bike and is designed to negotiate rough terrain and unpaved surfaces. The wheelbase is generally longer and, wider which makes it more stable. The rear wheels are generally highly cambered making it even more stable. The front wheels are connected with a tie-rod, but not always. Many off-road wheelchairs have hand operated, dynamic braking and active suspension systems.

Off-road wheelchair

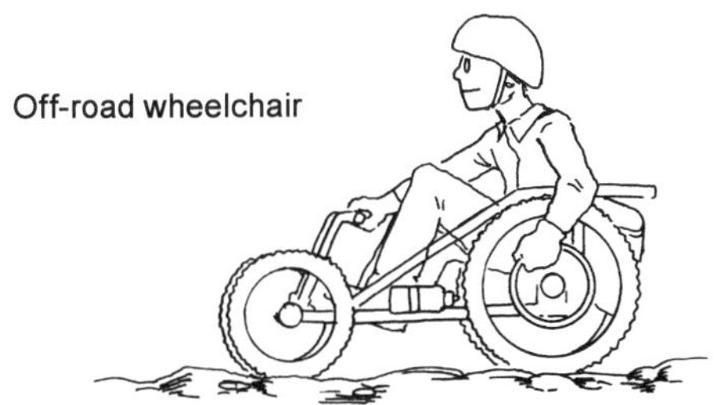

One arm drive wheelchairs

These chairs are designed for users that only have the use of one arm to both propel and steer the wheelchair. There are two types of one-arm drive wheelchairs One type has two handrims attached to one wheel. The outside handrim controls the opposite wheel and the inside hand-rim controls the wheel on the same side. With a collapsing scissor drive chair the wheelchair can still fold.

The other type has a lever to drive and steer the wheelchair. Using the left or right hand as ordered, the lever is pumped forward and backward to propel the wheelchair. Twisting the handgrip left or right turns the chair. Some one arm drive wheelchairs use a spring loaded bar that has to be removed from the wheelchair in order to fold the chair for transport.

Pool wheelchair

These chairs are transfer chairs used by a wheelchair user to roll down a ramp into a swimming pool. These chairs are designed to roll into the water and are often constructed of stainless steel or plastic. Most of these chairs have hard solid plastic seats and removable arm supports. They are most often self-propelled with push handles.

Quad rugby wheelchairs

These have a lowered seat height with significant seat dump for postural stability and have cambered rear wheels with a shorter wheelbase for the forward players. The chairs for defensive players have extended foot supports to block other players. The chairs have spoke protectors and a protective cage around the front of the wheelchair.

Racing wheelchair

A lightweight, three-wheeled wheelchair designed in an aerodynamic shape to maximize traveling speed. Used for training and racing events that take place on tracks or on roads.

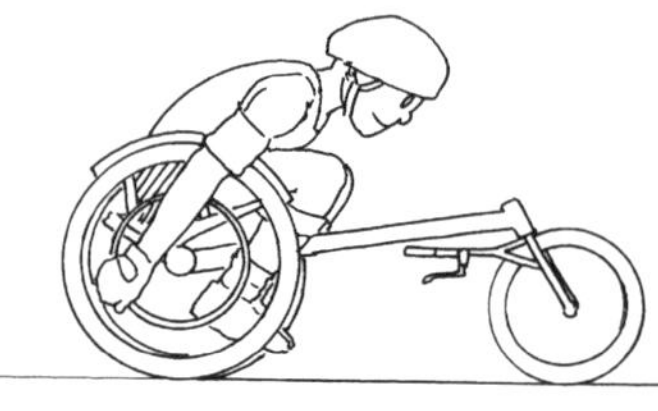

Racing wheelchair

Recliner wheelchairs

On a recliner chair, the backrest position is easily adjusted relative to the seat; such that when "fully reclined" the backrest and the seat are continuous in a horizontal position – allowing the rider to "lay down" or "stretch out".

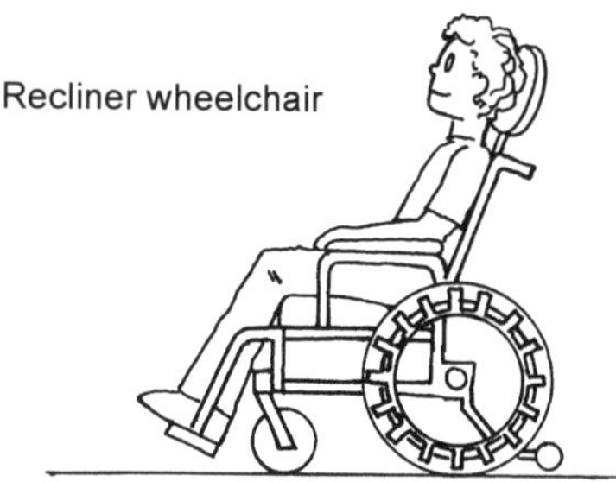

Recliner wheelchair

Recliner wheelchairs are most often used by people who use gravity to help balance their trunks, cannot maintain an upright sitting posture, have limited movement at their hips, or need to recline in order to relieve pressure from their buttocks. The rear wheels on recliner wheelchairs are further back, making the wheelchair more stable (harder to tip backwards). It also makes it harder to reach the handrims to propel. The wheelchair may have anti-tip devices installed to prevent the chair from tipping over backwards. Anti-tip devices are small-diameter wheels that attach at the back of the chair to provide additional rear stability.

Shower chair wheelchair

Shower chair wheelchairs are either stainless steel or plastic and are designed for toileting and showering. They usually have a commode style seat and can either be rolled over a toilet or used as a commode with the commode pail in place.

They are designed to roll into an accessible shower. Shower chair wheelchairs usually have standard wheel locks, and removable or swing away arm and foot supports. They are made in self-propelled and attendant propelled versions.

Standing wheelchair

These allow the user to achieve a standing position. Most standing wheelchairs are mobile in the sitting position and when they raise to the standing position are not mobile. Some are mobile in the standing position also. They are usually used to access various locations, but there are numerous physical benefits to standing, including: stretching of the muscles, loading the bones, draining the bladder fully, and allowing internal organs to change position from sitting.

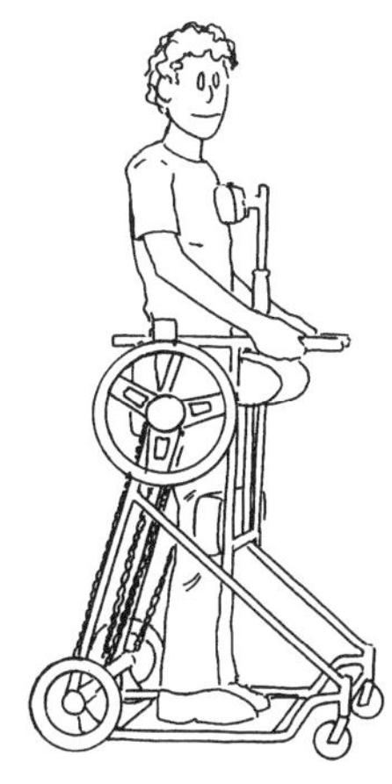

Standing wheelchair

Tennis wheelchair

This is designed for playing tennis and other racquet sports. Generally with significant rear wheel camber for increased lateral stability. The user general sits in a very compact position to reduce the moment of inertia for quicker turns. Tennis chairs usually have one or two front casters and sometimes a single anti-tip wheel in the rear.

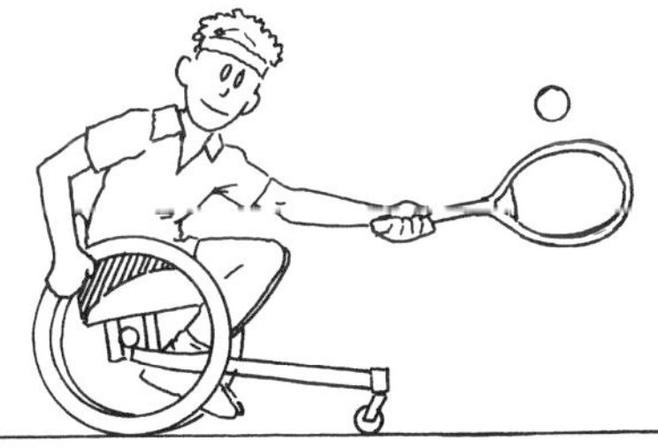

Tennis wheelchair

Tilt-in-space wheelchairs

These allow the user to change the orientation of the seat on the frame by allowing the entire seating system (the seat, back and foot support) to tilt back. This allows for a mechanical weight shift to provide increased postural stability and can provide an effective pressure relief. Tilt-in-space wheelchairs require a long wheelbase for stability. This decreases the maneuverability of the wheelchair.

Wheelchair Component Selection

Most manual wheelchairs feature these basic components:

- Rear wheels
- Front caster wheels
- Solid/pneumatic tires
- Arm supports
- Arm support panels or skirt guards
- Handrims
- Foot supports
- Wheel locks
- Sling or rigid back support
- Sling or rigid seat support

The materials, design, and adjustment of these components will affect your wheelchairs performance and fit. This training guide describes the proper adjustment and fitting of your wheelchair.

Rear wheels

Many types of rear wheels are available for manual wheelchairs. Most are either mag or spoke. Mag wheels are usually made from hard plastic and typically have only five or six molded ribs between the hub and wheel rim. Mag wheels are virtually maintenance-free and more durable than spoked wheels, but are usually heavier. There are now lighter weight and flexible fibers being used for spokes.

The spokes on a spoked wheel keep the wheel round. The quality of spoked wheels has improved; however, spokes can loosen, break, or fall out. If spokes break or fall out they must be replaced to keep the wheel round. Spokes should also be checked for their tension as uneven tension will also cause the wheel to go "out of round." The same wrench used to tighten bike wheel spokes can be used on wheelchair wheels. A good bike shop can usually help true your wheels to be round and planar with the spokes evenly tightened. The range of options in spoked wheels is quite large – reflected in the wide price range of spoked wheels. The goal is to find the diameter, size and tread pattern you want with the lightest weight and durability required to fit your lifestyle and propulsion demands.

The diameter of the rear wheels affect how your wheelchair performs. In the past, the standard rear wheel diameter has always been 24 inches. Now it is common to see 25-inch diameter rear wheels. Taller wheelchair users often prefer 26 or even 27-inch diameter wheels. Smaller rider's, those with shorter arms, may benefit from smaller wheels like 22". The wheel's size determines the handrim position in relation to your hands, affecting your ability to propel the chair efficiently, using less effort. You should be using the wheel size that is appropriate for your size, so people with longer arms (taller people) are often more comfortable and efficient pushing on larger wheels.

Larger wheels roll over obstacles and rough terrain easier and may improve wheeling efficiency for you.

Rear wheels with quick-release axles allow you to detach your rear wheels in a few seconds without tools for transport or storage.

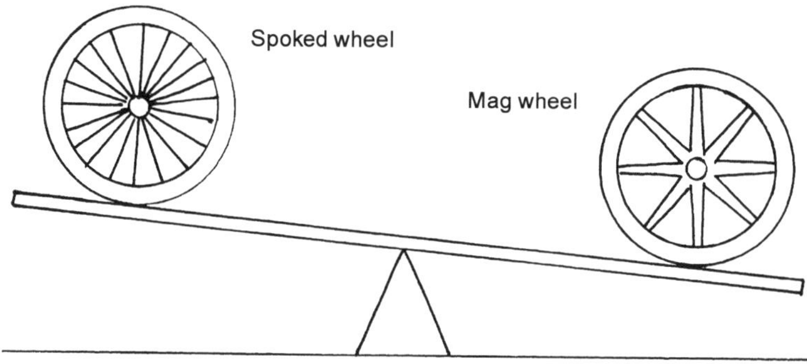

Rear tires

Rear tires for wheelchairs are either air-filled (pneumatic) or solid (flat-free or airless). Pneumatic tires require a specific air pressure to provide optimal performance. On uneven and outdoor surfaces, pneumatic tires usually give a more cushioned, smoother ride and are easier to propel than solid tires. If you only use your wheelchair on hard, smooth surfaces, solid, flat free, or semi pneumatic tires may make your wheelchair easier to propel. However, the tread on pneumatic tires tends to wear out more quickly than the tread on solid ones. If you have pneumatic tires, you may want to carry a patch kit, pump, and/or spare tire tube at all times to avoid being stranded by a flat. Pneumatic tire rims can be filled with solid inserts instead of tubes providing a tread to reduce slippage when wet while benefitting from the advantages of a maintenance free tire. Note that a flat free filler provides a firmer, stiffer ride than an air-filled tire. Some inserts take away some of the cushioning properties of air-filled inner tube tires.

Solid tires are filled with a foam core or another type of flat-free insert. Solid tires only need to be replaced for tread wear. Because solid tires are stiffer than pneumatic tires they usually have less shock absorbing capabilities and they give a bumpier ride over uneven surfaces. If you only use your wheelchair on smooth, hard surfaces, solid tires can make rolling your wheelchair easier.

Tire tread also affects your wheelchair's performance. Knobbier tires perform better on rough terrain because they provide more traction. The same knobby tread that grips so well also tracks more mud, snow, and dirt inside than smooth ones. Unless you plan to wear gloves and push on the tire, select knobby tires that do not have the knobs on the side where they will rub against your hands when using the handrims. Knobby tires also require more effort to propel over smooth surfaces than smooth tires. Smooth tires are more maneuverable over hard, flat surfaces, but make rolling over rough terrain more difficult.

Handrims

The handrim is usually attached to the wheel near the wheel's rim. A spacer on the bolt attaching the handrim to the wheel gives you room to grip the handrim with your fingers. You can use a shorter spacer to bring the handrim closer to the wheel. This narrows the overall wheelchair width but may make it more difficult to get a good grip on the handrim. If the space is too large, you may catch your thumb in the gap.

Hand rims are available in a variety of materials and styles. Metal handrims are sometimes difficult to use because they are slippery and get very cold, especially in winter. Rubber coated or textured handrims might improve your grip and allow you to push more strongly, but the extra friction will cause your hands to burn when going downhill. Because of this problem, coated handrim users usually wear gloves to push their wheelchairs. The coating can also wear off with repeated scraping against obstacles like wall corners and narrow doorways.

Handrims with projections can make it easier to push with less hand function. Handrim projections are often available angled more vertically or horizontally to accommodate different pushing styles.

Ergonomic handrims

A variety of ergonomic handrims are now available. Be sure to try them out. Choose ones that are comfortable for starting, stopping, and turning on flats or hills. Traditional handrims require a strong grip to push up a hill. When shopping for ergonomic handrims choose ones that minimize the amount of grip strength that is required to push your chair on soft surfaces and up hills. This will reduce the repetitive stress and strain on your hands over the long term. The addition of ergonomic handrims is perhaps the greatest improvement you can make to your existing or new wheelchair. Ergonomic handrims that are flexibly attached to the wheels will flex absorbing shock during propulsion and allow you to squeeze through narrow doorways as well.

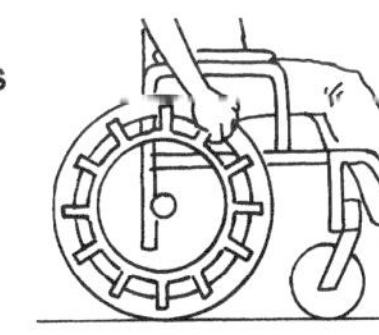
Handrim projections

Wheel locks

Wheel locks are sometimes just called brakes or parking brakes. Wheel locks are generally available in low- and high-mount versions and are selected when you order your chair. Low-mount wheel locks interfere less with your hand's movements but may be harder for some people to engage and disengage. Swing-away wheel locks (also known as scissor wheel locks) may be desirable since you can avoid hitting your thumbs on them when pushing directly on the tires. Some manufacturers have designed wheel locks that mount under the seat so they do not get in the way of pushing. Remember, locking the wheels, although very effective at stabilizing the chair in the right conditions, will not always keep your wheelchair from sliding if the ground is uneven, smooth, wet, or sloped.

You will have to adjust the mounting of your wheel locks after you change the rear wheel position, size, or type of tire so they will work effectively. If you use air-filled tires, the function of the wheel lock will change with the tire pressure. As your tire loses air, the wheel lock may slip. Check your owner's manual and follow the manufacturer's instructions to determine how far the wheel locks should penetrate into the tire when they are in the locked position.

Wheel locks are not running brakes that can be applied while you are moving to slow down the speed of your roll. However dynamic wheel locks are available for manual wheelchairs that can be used while traveling downhill. This type of brake serves as both a wheel lock and a dynamic wheel lock.

Front caster wheels

The two small wheels at the front of your wheelchair are called the caster wheels or casters. Caster wheels can swivel or pivot in all directions and improve your wheelchair's maneuverability. Caster stem housings connect the caster wheels to your wheelchair frame.

Many different types of caster wheels with a range of performance features are available. Small, hard wheels (like rollerblade wheels) can improve maneuverability on hard, flat surfaces but tend to catch in the cracks and crevices of rough surfaces. Larger pneumatic caster wheels are less likely to catch in crevices or on obstacles and handle better over rough terrain but are harder to pivot on almost all surfaces.

Solid rubber or plastic caster wheels usually give a rougher ride than pneumatic caster wheels because they have little shock-absorbing ability. Some users do not like the vibration that occurs using solid rubber caster or plastic caster wheels.

Semi-pneumatic or pneumatic caster wheels give a smoother ride than solid caster wheels and roll over all sorts of obstacles outdoors; however, pneumatic caster wheels have more rolling resistance on hard flat surfaces and can go flat.

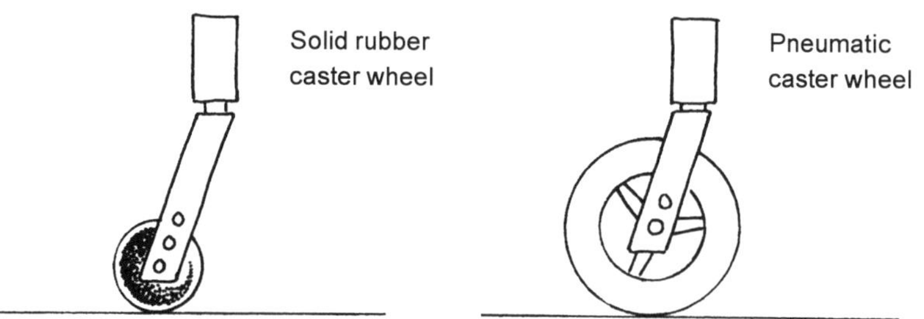

Arm supports

The preference for arm supports (often called armrests) varies. Many wheelchair users feel they cannot live without arm supports. Other users do not want arm supports at all. Your personal preference, level of function, and balance will determine whether you want or need arm supports and will impact the type of arm support that will work best for you. Arm supports can provide additional support if you have limited trunk balance and can act as side-to-side stability anchors when you reach sideways. However, many manual wheelchair users do not use arm supports because they may get in the way during propulsion, weight shifts and transfers. They also add to the overall weight of your wheelchair making it somewhat more cumbersome to manage. Transfers in and out of your wheelchair and weight shifts may require more strength and balance without arm supports. If you choose to use arm supports, make sure the style, placement, and height does not interfere with propelling your wheelchair. Your arm supports should be used for resting and should allow you to place your elbows slightly forward of your shoulders when resting your arms.

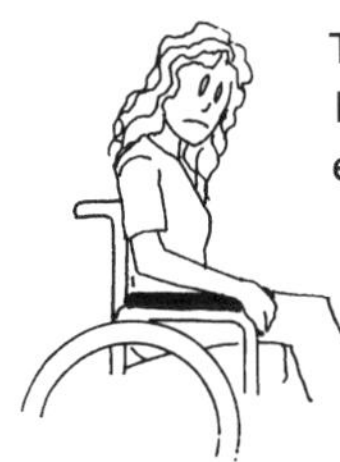

This arm support is too low and does not provide enough arm support.

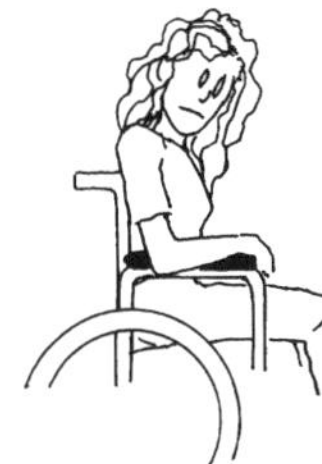

This arm support is too high and pushes the rider's arms up into her shoulders.

Verify Correct Seating Dimensions

Seat width

Your wheelchair seat should be as narrow as possible without touching your hipbones or thigh bones. If the seat is too narrow, it could cause a pressure ulcer. If the seat is too wide, you might have difficulty propelling your chair and getting through doorways. A wide chair might also cause you to lean to the side when you sit or propel, which could lead to the development of a spinal deformity like scoliosis.

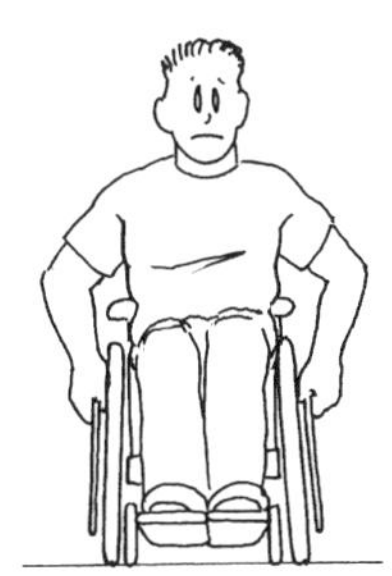

This seat is too narrow.

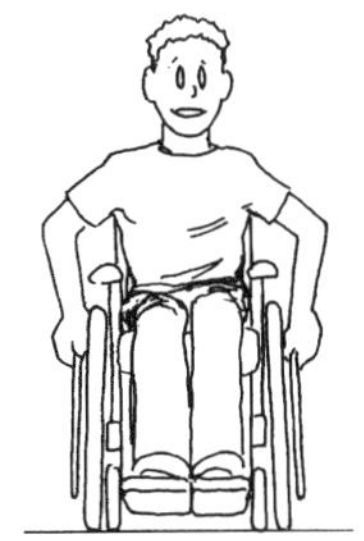

This seat is just right.

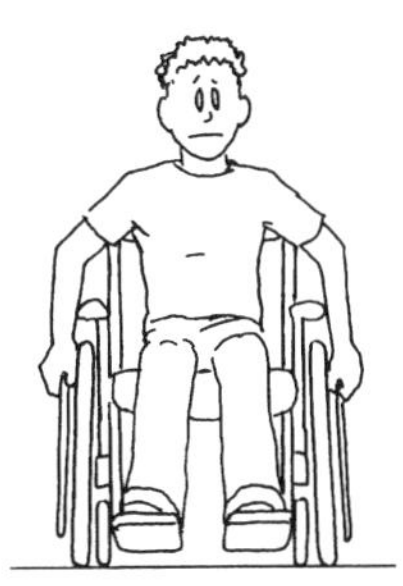

This seat is too wide.

There should be about half an inch of space on either side of your hips. The space gives you a little room to move and tuck in your clothing. Seat width affects the overall width of your wheelchair.

Seat depth

The right seat depth is essential for providing the right amount of support under your thighs. If the seat is too shallow, you will experience more pressure on your sitting area, and you could develop pressure ulcers. If the seat is too deep, you will be unable to move all the way against the back of the chair and you will end up slouching backward. A seat that is too deep could interfere with circulation to your legs and cause pressure ulcers behind your knees.

The correct seat depth typically permits about one inch of space between the front edge of the cushion and the back of your knees. The distance needed may be larger if you regularly use your hands to lift your legs, or if you propel your wheelchair with your legs and feet.

If the seat upholstery or seat is too long:

- Talk to a seating specialist about shortening the upholstery or the solid seat beneath your seat cushion.

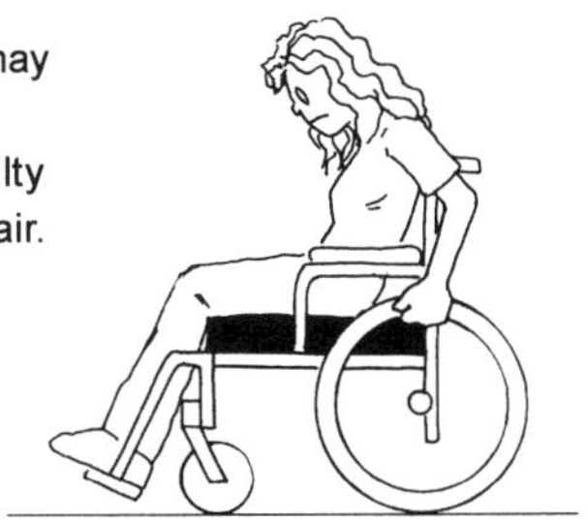

This seat is too long. Pressure may develop behind your knees and thighs, and you may have difficulty sitting all the way back in the chair.

If the seat cushion is too long:

- Get a shorter cushion or if possible, modify the rear corners of the cushion so it fits farther back on the seat support surface of your wheelchair.
- Move your back support further forward or get a thicker back support, which will move you forward in your seat and shorten the overall seat depth. Remember that this might also change your position in relation to the handrims, so you might have to make other adjustments too.
- Another option is to move the seat cushion back. Sometimes the cushion will even slide under the back support. Make sure your buttocks are still positioned correctly on the cushion.

If the seat is too short:

- Move the back support back if you can. This will allow you to move farther back in your wheelchair, lengthening the seat depth and making room for a longer seat cushion. Remember that this might change your position in relation to your handrims so you may need to make other adjustments when you change the position of the back support.
- Use a longer seat cushion supported over the front edge of the seat upholstery by a firm board or sheet of stiff plastic.

If the seat cushion is too short:

- Get a longer cushion.

This seat and seat cushion is too short. Pressures will be higher on your sitting area.

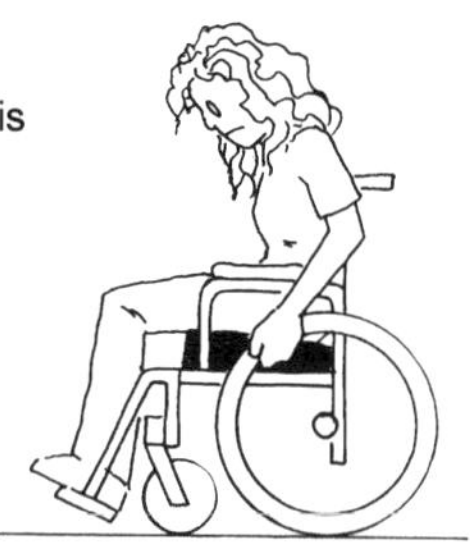

Wheelchair Setup

When determining the dimensions for a new wheelchair, refer to A guide to Wheelchair Selection (Axelson, Minkel & Chesney, 2006) for guidance. If you already have a wheelchair that has a suitable seat width and depth, adjustments can be made to the chair to make it a better fit. Below is a prioritized list of adjustments that should be considered.

Seat cushion

The seat cushion that you need to sit on has to be considered first, before all of the other adjustments on your wheelchair can be considered. Every wheelchair user that is sitting in a wheelchair for extended periods of time is going to want to sit on some type of seat cushion even if the cushion is just a simple 1 or 2 inch foam cushion. For wheelchair users without sensation or with difficulty moving, a pressure relieving cushion is going to be an important consideration. Generally the more pressure relief the taller the cushion is going to be but this does not necessarily mean that your sitting bones are going to be higher off the sling seating. When making measurements for a wheelchair, it is typically best to make all of the measurements while sitting on the seat cushion that will be used in the wheelchair. Some users like to sit on different cushions depending on what they are doing. If a sport chair is being used with one type of seat cushion and an everyday wheelchair is being used with a different seat cushion for everything else, each wheelchair will need to be set up and adjusted while sitting on the specific seat cushion that will be used for the specific wheelchair. Some users have two different types of cushions that they sit on that are different heights for the same wheelchair. This can be accommodated by using an insert beneath the lower height seat cushion so that the height of the seat cushion is the same as the higher seat cushion.

Adjusting the seat angle

Moving the rear axle mounting location up will lower the rear of your wheelchair frame which causes the chair to tip back and lowers the seat height. Then the caster stem housings will need to be adjusted to a vertical position (perpendicular to the ground) so that the chair will roll correctly. This adjustment is possible with most higher end “rehab” wheelchair models. Occasionally there is a vertical adjustment for the caster stem housings to lower the front of your wheelchair frame as well. In other cases it is possible to move the caster wheel upward in the front caster forks. Another possible change is to use a shorter front caster fork or a shorter caster stem bolt. Using a smaller diameter front caster wheel is another way to lower the front end of your wheelchair. Moving the rear axle down will raise your wheelchair frame in the rear, which will raise the seat height in the rear but will cause the seat support surface to tilt forward.

After adjusting the vertical position of the rear wheels, you may also have to change the height and/or angle of the caster wheels to maintain your desired seat plane angle. Make sure the caster stem housings are vertical (perpendicular to the ground) so that the chair will roll correctly.

Hemi-height wheelchair has a lower seat height.
This seat is lower with a high rear axle position.

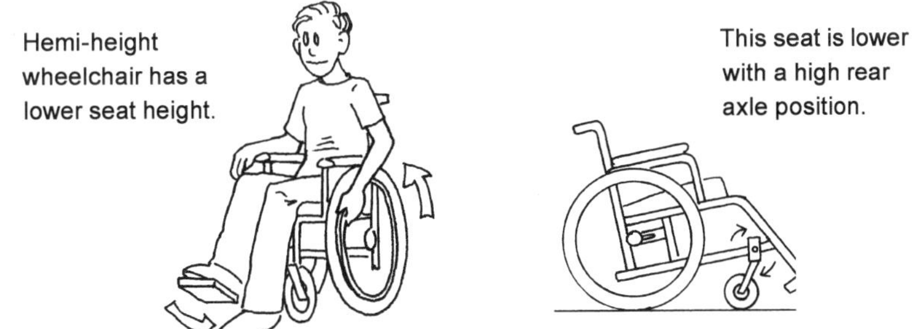

If you adjust your vertical position in your wheelchair via the seat rather than the wheel axle, you will not have to readjust the caster stem housings when you change the seat and back position. This adjustment is only possible on some wheelchair models.

Adjusting the back support height

The back support height should be comfortable and provide good lower back support. A lower back support lets you move your arms and upper body more. If needed, a higher back support provides more upper-body support.

The back posts or push handles should not interfere with arm movements while you are wheeling. They may be adjustable in height. Check with your supplier or the user manual for further information. Many wheelchair users do not like push handles since they get in the way and they seem to encourage well-meaning people to push the wheelchair without asking. Fold-down, push handles are available on some wheelchairs. They can be put in place when you need them and folded down when they are not needed. Back supports are also available without push handles but if you sometimes need help from someone else to propel or maneuver your chair, push handles make it much easier for the assistant.

Adjusting the back support angle

Your back support angle should provide a comfortable sitting posture while you are upright in the wheelchair. The back support angle should not cause you to slump, curl your shoulders, hold your head forward for balance, or cause you to slide out of your seat.

The angle formed by the seat and the back support is called the seat-to-back angle. The seat-to-back angle greater than 90°

is an open angle, while an angle smaller (tighter) than 90° is a closed angle. An open angle lets you use gravity to help balance your trunk. People who cannot flex well at the hips often use an open seat-to-back support angle. However, an open angle may cause people to slide out of their chairs. The open angle may also change your position in relation to the handrims making your wheelchair harder to propel.

A closed angle cradles the body in the curve of the seat, holding you in place and often reducing leg spasticity. Some people combine this with a higher rear axle position which lowers the back of the seat creating even more of a cradle. This is sometimes called seat dumping. People with high spinal cord injuries and very poor trunk balance prefer a more closed seat-to-back angle for enhanced trunk stability. Not all wheelchair users can tolerate a more closed (or tighter) seat-to-back angle which requires more hip flexion. Be sure you have sufficient range of motion at the hips if you are considering closing your seat-to-back angle. This can be helpful to people with limited fore aft trunk movement and stability as it provides the needed support by changing the direction of the force of gravity while increasing maneuverability by keeping the shoulders in a better position to push the wheels.

Adjusting the seat surface height, leg support, and foot clearance

Your seat height and leg support length and angle are interdependent and must be determined together. Your seat height determines the vertical space available for your legs thereby determining the degree of leg angle necessary to accommodate the length of your legs. Inversely, your leg angle can determine how high your seat must be to accommodate your leg length, leg angle, and your feet on the foot supports. It is important that the seat is high enough for your foot supports to clear obstacles and low enough for your knees to fit under tables. According to the Americans with Disabilities Act Accessibility Guidelines, standard tables or counters should have knee clearance spaces at least 27 inches high.

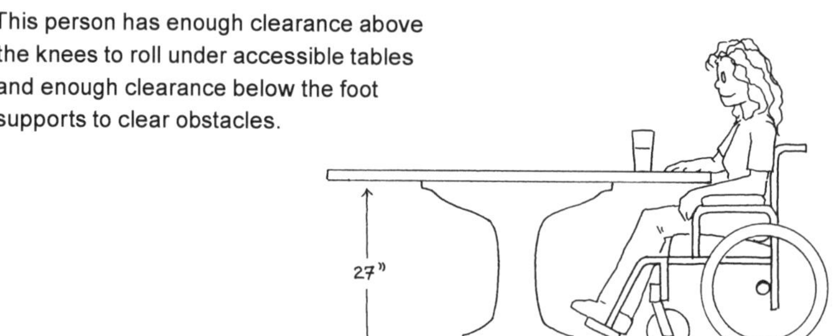

This person has enough clearance above the knees to roll under accessible tables and enough clearance below the foot supports to clear obstacles.

Your leg angle will impact your comfort and the length of your footprint. A larger angle from the bottom of the seat to the back of the calves will allow greater foot support clearance and/or a lower seat height. This means that your feet will be out further in front of you which makes your overall length longer and might make maneuvering in small spaces more difficult. Some people will choose to have their legs angled under the chair. This reduces the length of your footprint and provides a "sportier" look, but will decrease your stability and may impact the blood circulation in your legs and feet.

There are factors that can be altered to help accommodate the necessary seat height, leg angle, and ground clearance. These factors include the vertical rear wheel height, the caster height, the axel position, and your seat cushion thickness. Larger rear wheels and front casters will raise the chair higher off the ground. Smaller rear wheels and front casters will lower the chair. Lowering the rear wheel axle position will raise the rear of your wheelchair higher off the ground while raising the axle position will bring the rear of the wheelchair closer to the ground. You can increase the seat cushion thickness to raise the seat height by adding padding or a solid insert under the cushion. You can decrease cushion thickness to lower the seat height.

Making changes to your axel position and wheel height will change your position in relation to the handrims which may make it harder or easier to propel your wheelchair. Lowering the seat height will make it easier to reach the handrims, which might provide more power when you propel your wheelchair. If you are too low in relation to the handrims but need the lower seat height, you can replace the rear wheels with smaller diameter ones. You can also use smaller rear wheels if you want the seat height to be even lower.

There are other ways to raise your wheelchair seat height. The height of some wheelchair seat support surfaces are adjustable and can be raised to accommodate leg length and leg clearance. Seat supports with extensions can also be installed to raise the seat higher.

If your legs are long, you might have to compromise between sitting comfort and leg clearance. It is more important for you to fit properly and comfortably in your wheelchair than to be able to roll under all tables. If you need more clearance under a table at home or work you could raise the table up higher. You can place a layer of plywood beneath the base or between the tabletop and the base. If the table has individual legs you can make blocks of wood with shallow holes on the tops of them to keep the blocks positioned under the table legs. Make sure the table is secure and will not slide off whatever you use to raise the table up. A higher seat is also useful for people who have difficulty standing up from or sitting down onto low surfaces.

Foot supports

After determining your seat height and leg angle, adjust the positioning of your foot supports. You should have your cushion, back support, and other positioning aids in place when adjusting your foot supports. Don't forget to put your normal shoes on; sole height affects your leg positioning. Make sure you are seated upright against the back of the chair. When adjusting the foot supports:

- Make sure you have clearance of two inches underneath the foot plates so your foot plates do not get caught on small obstacles in the roadway.
- Also have clearance for your knees under desks and tables.
- Some experienced users ride with less ground clearance so that if the wheelchair tips forward on a level surface, the foot supports themselves will prevent the chair from tipping over forward.

If you do not have enough clearance, you might need to readjust the seat plane angle and height. When your feet are supported at the correct height by your foot supports, your thighs should rest in a balanced manner on your cushion. Foot supports that are too high can lead to little or no weight under your thighs (especially near your knees) and cause excessive weight under your sitting bones, the ischial tuberosities, which could lead to pressure sore development. You might need to compromise on your knee height and how easily you can roll under tables without hitting, in order to get the best leg support.

Some wheelchairs can be ordered with a steeper footrest angle at the front, allowing your legs to be tucked further under the chair versus having your feet out in front of your wheelchair. This shortens the overall length and may make it easier for you to maneuver your wheelchair in tight spaces.

Swing-away foot supports can be moved out of the way or removed. When you take your feet off the foot supports and swing them out of the way or remove them, you should be able to get closer to obstacles but, your feet will be dangling. If they reach the ground, you may still get the support you need to hold your balance while sitting close to a desk or table, but if you need your feet and legs to be well supported in order to have trunk balance, removing your feet from the foot supports may cause you to lose your balance. Removing or swinging away the foot supports may be necessary for you to perform safe transfers to and from your wheelchair.

Adjusting rear wheel camber

Camber is the off-vertical tilt of the rear wheels. It widens the distance between the bottoms of the propulsion wheels and narrows the distance between the tops of the wheels. Wheel camber increases side-to-side and forward stability. Camber also increases your wheelchair's overall width, which may make it difficult to roll through narrow doorways. Increasing wheel camber may also make your seat width narrower so make sure your hips are not rubbing or squeezed. Follow the owner's manual instructions to adjust wheel camber.

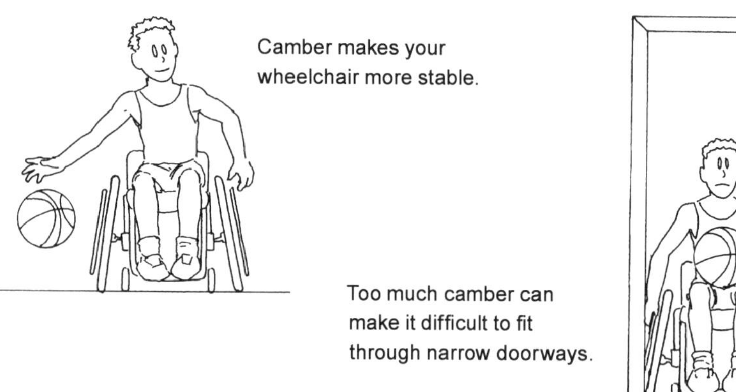

Camber makes your wheelchair more stable.

Too much camber can make it difficult to fit through narrow doorways.

When adjusting the camber of your rear wheels, be careful not to set them toed in or out. Toed out means the front edge of the rear wheels are pointed outward away from your feet. Toed in means the front edge of your rear wheels are pointed inward, toward each other and your feet. Setting the wheels to toe in or toe out will make your wheelchair more difficult to propel and causes the tires to wear unevenly.

Adjusting the rear wheel axle horizontally

Next, set the horizontal position of the rear wheel to meet your stability requirements. Surprisingly, a completely stable wheelchair is not always desirable. As with many vehicles, including cars, bicycles, and motorcycles, a wheelchair that is less stable in the rearward direction is also easier to maneuver. Your chair will provide the best performance if you position the rear axle as far forward as you can while maintaining your balance comfortably during all types of activities. Rear wheels that are set too far forward may interfere with the movement of the front caster wheels while making the wheelbase extremely short and your wheelchair unstable. You will tip over backwards too easily if you set the rear axle too far forward for your ability and the environments where you use your wheelchair.

Moving the rear axle in the fore/aft direction (forward or backward) changes the location of the center of gravity with respect to the rear wheels. The more forward the axle is positioned, the less weight will be over the front caster wheels. This will make the chair easier to tip back and pop into a wheelie, but will also make it more difficult to push up a hill without tipping backward. It is much easier to maneuver over obstacles and turn around in small spaces in a wheelie (Section 1.9 has more information about wheelies.)

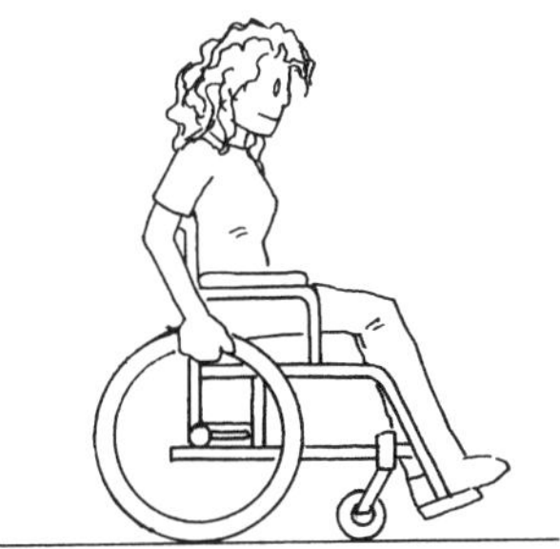

The rear wheel is far back and the center of gravity is forward of the rear axle position. This makes the wheelchair very stable in the rearward direction and difficult to pop into a wheelie. It also may make the whole wheelchair longer and more difficult to navigate in small spaces.

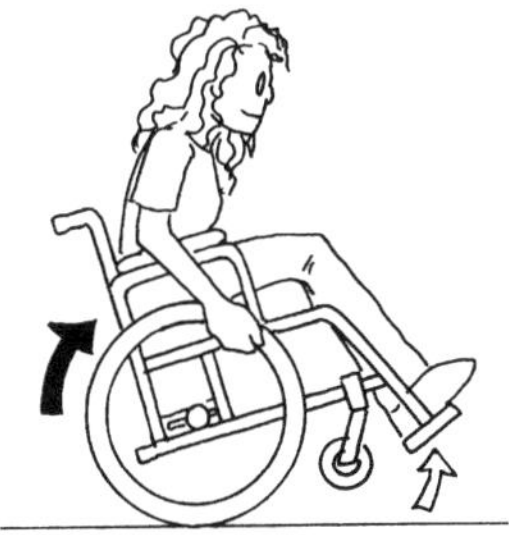

The rear wheel is forward and the center of gravity is closer to the rear axle position. This makes your wheelchair tip easier in the rearward direction and easier to pop into a wheelie. It also may shorten the overall length of your wheelchair.

If you know how to hold a "wheelie" – balance the chair on the rear wheels only – you may want to start the rear wheel adjustment about 2" forward of the back posts. Test the stability of the chair. With either someone behind you to "spot", or by having an anti-tipping device on the chair, give the chair a push forward, are you comfortable with the response? If the chair tips back to far, or too fast; consider moving the wheels back slightly. If you are comfortable with the chair's response, you may want to move the wheel further forward to find the spot where you are uncomfortable, then move it back slightly. True wheelie performance begins at the edge of your comfort zone.

Test drive each new setup by going up a standard ramp with a spotter to make sure the position of the rear wheel axle will not cause your wheelchair to tip over backward.

Adjusting the caster stem housing

Your caster stem housings should be perpendicular to the ground. If they are not, your front caster wheels may become afflicted with "shopping cart syndrome" and flutter when you propel your chair. This may also make it difficult to turn your wheelchair or change direction. Use a book or carpenter's angle to make sure the caster stem housing is perpendicular to the ground. Consult your owner's manual for detailed instructions on how to adjust the caster stem housing angle.

Section 1.3

Asking for Help

Public awareness of access issues is constantly improving. Strides are being made every day toward the goal of universal access for people with disabilities. However, situations will still arise where you need help. Everyone needs help now and then. The need for assistance varies from situation to situation and from person to person. It can be difficult for some people to know when they should ask for help. Some ask more often than they need, while others fail to ask at all. Some people have difficulty asking for help because they are embarrassed or they just do not know how to explain what they need. The more you practice asking for help, the easier it will get and the better you will get at explaining what you need.

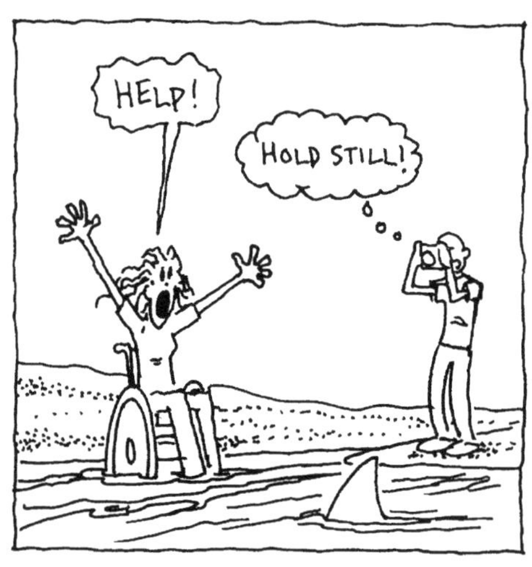

Defining "Assistance"

"Assistance" has many meanings. You may need help to push your wheelchair because a shoulder injury has temporarily made propulsion difficult and painful. You may need help reaching a package of corn chips on a high shelf at the store. You may need help being lifted up stairs, over loose gravel, up a steep hill, or any number of other situations that are difficult or unsafe for you to do by yourself. The following are different levels of skill that may require assistance:

Independent Skills – Actions you can perform without help.

Supervised/Assisted Skills – Actions you can participate in but are uncomfortable doing completely alone. You might need occasional help or someone nearby "just in case." Being able to ask for and instruct others how to help is very important.

Dependent Skills – Actions you can only perform with a lot of help.

Who Can Help?

A variety of people are available to give you assistance when you need it. These roles vary depending on the situation and your ability:

Spotter – This is a person who stands nearby to help if you need it. Recruit a spotter when learning a new skill and when you are not confident of your own abilities. This person is usually there to keep you from tipping over backward or falling forward out of your wheelchair. It is up to you to decide when you are uncomfortable with a maneuver and would like to use a spotter. You might even need more than one person to help when learning a new skill.

Assistant – A spotter becomes an assistant when you know you will need help or require more than an occasional hand. Assisting often involves pushing or lifting your wheelchair in some capacity (such as up a flight of stairs or over a curb that is too high to cross independently). An assistant might also be asked to perform other tasks such as picking up items you drop or getting things you cannot reach. In many cases, the assistant is a passerby who is willing to help. Sometimes, an assistant is hired and trained by the wheelchair user. These assistants are often referred to as personal care assistants (PCAs) or attendants.

Personal Care Assistant (PCA)

If you need help frequently or at regular times during the day, you may want to hire a PCA. Some wheelchair users find it difficult to ask family members or friends to help because they feel they are burdening them. Relationships with family members or friends may become strained if they always feel responsible for helping you.

A potential advantage of a hired assistant is that he or she can help you with personal tasks that you might not want to ask a friend or family member to help with, such as bowel and bladder care. Hired assistants are generally not as emotionally involved with you and since they are hired to help, it might be easier for you to ask for help and not feel like you are burdening someone. It is the job of a hired assistant to provide the help you need in a given situation. You can train your personal assistant to do things the way you want. If the arrangement doesn't work out, you also have the freedom to replace the PCA.

Family and friends

Family and friends with whom you spend most of your time will need to spot or assist you on some occasions. It can be valuable to rely on people you are comfortable with when feeling strong emotions you don't want to express in front of strangers. Do not assume family members or friends will always be comfortable helping you. Be sure to ask if they are willing to help. Make sure they know not to help you unless you request assistance. You probably have a good idea of which friends and family you can trust as assistants based on your familiarity with their personalities.

Coworkers or acquaintances

Coworkers or friendly acquaintances can also make good assistants when you need help at work. If you are on good terms with a coworker, you may be comfortable casually asking for assistance (for example, "Hi, can you give me a push over this threshold? Thanks!"). You will also have to be the judge of whether you are asking too many people for help or asking for help too often. If that is the case, you may want to meet with a physical or occupational therapist who to can teach you the skills you need in order to be more independent. People you meet after your injury may be more comfortable with you as a wheelchair user than friends or family still making the adjustment to your new circumstances.

Strangers

When you are alone, situations may arise where you need a stranger's assistance. For example, you may have dropped your car keys where you cannot reach them. In this case, you may need to ask someone you do not know for help. Alternatively, you may be out with a friend and find yourself in a situation where the assistance of a second person is necessary or your friend might be unable to or uncomfortable with helping you. For example, you may need an additional person to help lift the front end of your wheelchair up some stairs.

How to Ask for Help

How you ask for help will vary from situation to situation. Ask for assistance in a way that allows the person to comfortably decline. Practice asking for assistance with a companion, acting as a stranger. This will help you learn how to ask strangers for assistance as well as teach your companion to help only when necessary. This type of practice also helps you learn how to instruct others to safely assist you.

Remember that there are many valid reasons for people to decline to help you. Some people have disabilities that are not visible, such as arthritis or heart disease, and they may be reluctant to disclose their condition to you. Other people's beliefs or customs may also prohibit them from assisting you. Other people may just be afraid they might hurt you.

Accept refusals to help gracefully. After all, you do not want help from a person who feels uncomfortable with the task because their apprehension can increase the risk of injury for both of you.

Consider the following before asking a stranger for help:

- Do not ask for assistance from anyone you think might be a threat.
- Consider the people around you, and approach the ones who look prepared to provide some physical assistance.
- Body size is unimportant when performing most assisting skills. Do not assume a smaller person is not strong enough to help you.
- Ask for assistance from people involved in activities similar to your own. For example, if you are shooting baskets in the park and lose the basketball in a bush, ask another ball player for assistance.
- If you enjoy challenging environments such as hiking trails, remember that this type of environment attracts a lot of people who, like yourself, are looking for an adventure. They may see helping you as yet another challenge and be very eager to assist.

Ask the jogger for assistance rather than the man in the suit. The person in the workout clothes is less likely to worry about getting dirty or wrinkled.

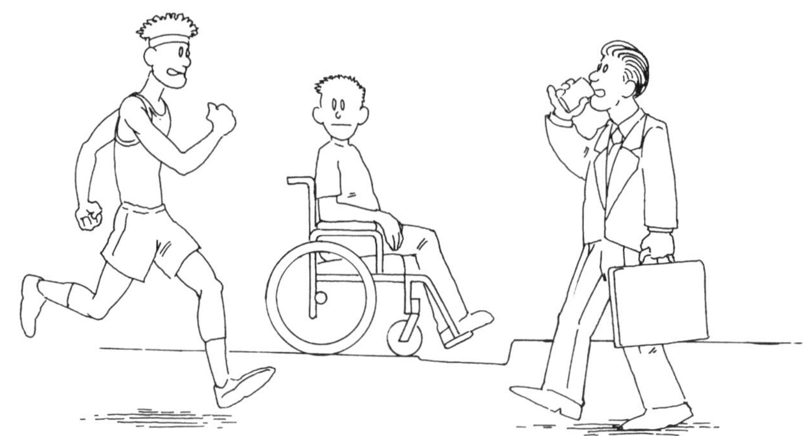

- If there are few people around and you know you will need assistance soon (for example, there is a curb around the corner), ask someone if they would be willing to follow you to the place where you will need help.
- Try "Do you mind giving me a hand up this curb?" or "Could you help me down this steep curb ramp? I can talk you through exactly what I need you to do."

Be clear and concise when giving instructions. Most of the skills in this manual include instructions you can give an assistant.

- You are in charge. Instruct your assistant not to do anything unless you specifically ask.
- (Read Section 5.1 for more information about protecting the back. Make sure friends and family who frequently assist you read that chapter also.)
- Tell your assistant where to stand.
- Indicate how to hold onto your wheelchair. (For example, "Please do not lift from the foot support because it might break off. Hold the frame next to my knees instead.")
- Give body mechanics instructions (for example, "Bend at your knees and keep your back straight.")
- Always instruct your assistant to move on your count of three to coordinate the efforts of all parties.
- Remember to thank your assistant for the help.

Describing Safe Body Mechanics

Since your spotter or assistant is being nice and helping you out, protect her/him by pointing out safe body positioning and mechanics. Section 5.1 contains additional information on safe body mechanics for helpers.

Always remind your helper to:

- Bend at the knees, not at the waist.
- Use legs for strength rather than the weaker muscles of the back or arms. This will help prevent back strain.
- Keep knees bent, not locked straight.
- Never twist at the waist. Instead, keep the torso facing the same direction as the hips and move the feet around to turn. This will help prevent back strain.
- Maintain a straight back. Hunching over or rounding the shoulders can cause back strain.
- Keep breathing. Sometimes people hold their breath when they are involved in physical activity. When you hold your breath, you are more likely to tense your muscles. Tense muscles are significantly more prone to strain.

When You Do Not Want or Need Assistance

Who says human nature isn't inherently good? You will find that some people will try to help you even when you haven't asked. While such intentions may be virtuous, their actions can be very frustrating and, at times, even dangerous. An unexpected push may catch you off balance and cause you to fly out of your wheelchair.

Decline their premature efforts by saying something like, "Thanks, but I'd like to do this myself" or "Thank you, but it is actually easier for me to do this without assistance." More aggressive good Samaritans may need to be deterred by a sharper directive such as, "Please don't grab my wheelchair."

You may have to be assertive when telling people not to help.

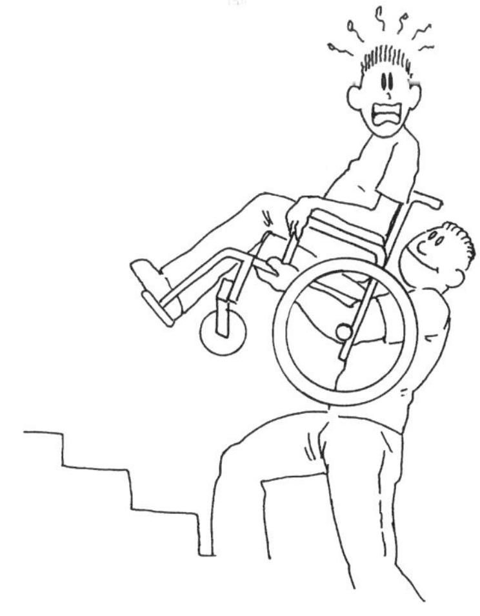

Section 1.4

Learning Your Limits

Riding at different speeds, traveling up and down hills, negotiating varying surfaces, and picking your way through assorted obstacles will affect your stability. It is important that you learn the limits of what you can do in a safe environment. When you are trying new things, make sure you have a spotter with you. Sometimes you can perform more advanced skills or roll over rougher terrain by shifting your weight to keep your balance. Before you try shifting your weight with your wheelchair moving, try it when your wheelchair is still. After you see how far you can lean with your wheelchair not moving, try shifting your weight while rolling in a variety of environments and over a variety of surfaces.

When testing your capabilities and trying out new things, avoid falls by practicing with a spotter. (Section 3.1 discusses techniques for falling and getting up.) As you experience what happens when you hit an obstacle, come to an abrupt halt, or propel down a ramp, you will learn how it affects your balance and when to ask for help. Always ask for assistance in situations that you know will exceed your limits.

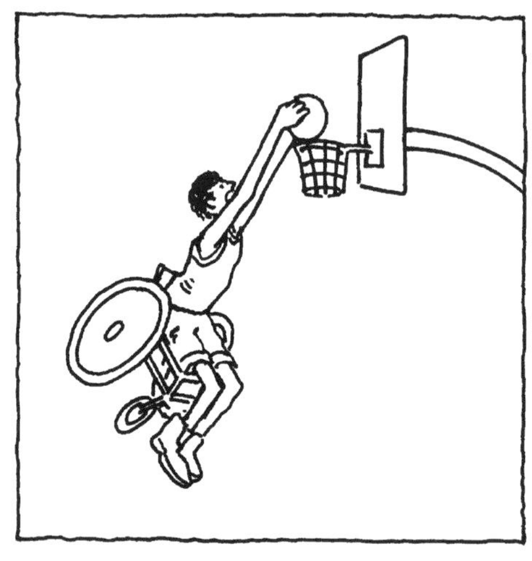

Shifting Your Weight Forward (Leaning Forward)

Shifting your weight forward can help you avoid tipping over backward when your wheelchair is in the wheelie position or going uphill. Your ability to lean forward depends on your balance and strength. You may be able to lean from your hips, chest, or perhaps with only your head. Lean forward when:

- Popping a wheelie (if you want your front casters to come up as high as possible)
- Going forward up hills and ramps
- Climbing curbs and stairs forward
- Descending curbs and stairs backward

- Your front wheels (casters) are going forward across thresholds and other obstacles (shift your weight back as the rear wheels cross the obstacle)
- Going up an escalator forward
- Going down an escalator backward

Forward weight shift technique

- When necessary, lean or bend forward into the slope.
- Only lean as far forward as is necessary to maintain your balance.
- When you are learning how far you can safely lean, start with your wheelchair in a stable position and position your caster wheels in the forward trailing position by wheeling backward for a short distance before you practice (see Section 1.5). This will make your wheelchair more stable.

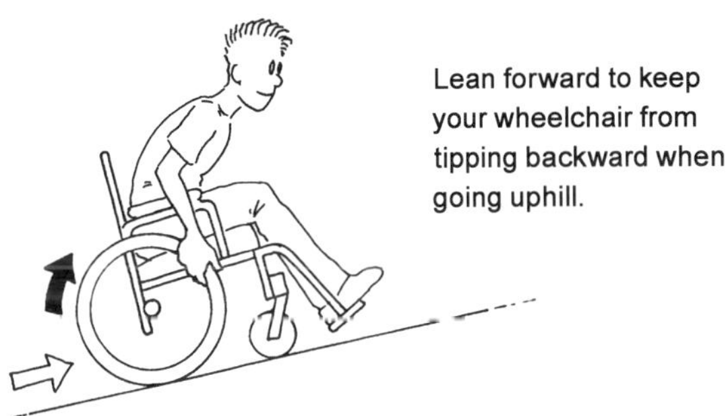

Lean forward to keep your wheelchair from tipping backward when going uphill.

How a spotter can help

- Stand behind the wheelchair user with their hands close to the push handles or pull straps.
- Keep the wheelchair user from tipping backward.

Shifting Your Weight Backward

Shifting your weight backward can prevent you from falling forward when your wheelchair is angled downward in the forward direction, such as when you are headed downhill. Your ability to lean back will depend on your upper-body strength and the height of your wheelchair back. The lower the chair back, the farther you can lean back. Many types of back support inserts are now available for manual wheelchairs. For stability, an adjustable back support would be moved back or loosened when going downhill and tightened while moving forward to go uphill.

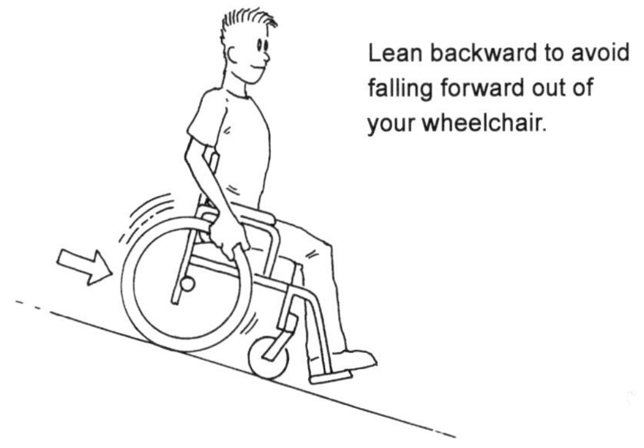

Lean backward to avoid falling forward out of your wheelchair.

Lean backward when:

- Popping a wheelie (if you want your front casters to come up as little as possible)
- When you need to push your front casters over a small threshold or obstacle
- Traveling down hills and ramps
- You are rolling backwards over a threshold or other obstacle

Backward weight shift technique

- When necessary, lean backward into the slope.
- Only lean as far back as is necessary.

How a spotter can help

- Stand to one side of the wheelchair user.
- Prevent the wheelchair user from falling forward by positioning a hand near his/her shoulder or in front of their chest.

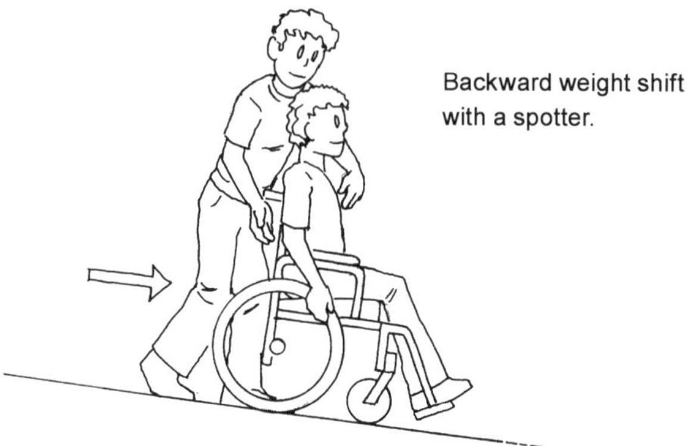

Backward weight shift with a spotter.

Sideways Weight Shift Technique

Many surfaces slope to the side including sidewalks and hillsides. Your wheelchair could tip over to the side if the slope is too steep. If you go up or down a ramp or other slope on a bit of an angle, even that side slope could cause your wheelchair to tip. Sometimes you can lean in the uphill direction to keep you and your wheelchair more stable on side slopes. Use an inclinometer (available in hardware stores or available as an application for many smart phones) or similar angle finding device to measure the angle of the slope on which you lose your stability. In this way, you can learn what the maximum slope you can negotiate looks like.

When necessary:

- Lean slightly toward the uphill slope.
- Only lean as far to the side as necessary.

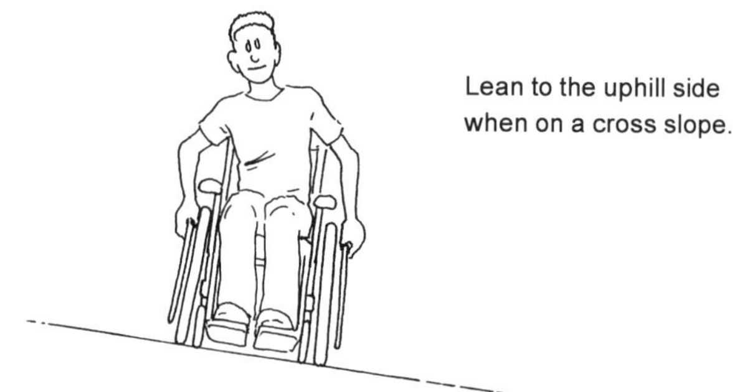

Lean to the uphill side when on a cross slope.

How a spotter can help

- Stand behind the wheelchair user with a hand near the rider's shoulder on the downhill side of the slope.
- Catch the rider at the shoulder if he or she begins to tip or fall out of their wheelchair.

Section 1.5

Caster Trail

Caster wheel position plays a major role in the stability of your wheelchair. Lengthening the wheelbase by reversing the caster wheel trail makes your wheelchair more stable. This is called the forward trailing position, meaning that most of the caster is forward of the caster housing. When your wheelchair is stopped and the casters are in this position, the overall length of your wheelchair is longer and therefore more stable. When you roll forward, the caster trails in the rearward position. When your wheelchair is stopped and the casters are in this position, the overall length of your wheelchair is shorter and is less stable. If you try to reach forward when the casters are trailed rearward like this, you may tip forward. When you turn to the left or right, especially in tight environments, the casters turn and trail to the side. If you pay attention to the position of your caster wheels when you are rolling, especially when traveling over obstacles and in tight environments, you may be able to avoid getting the casters caught in crevices that could stop your wheelchair abruptly and pitch you forward.

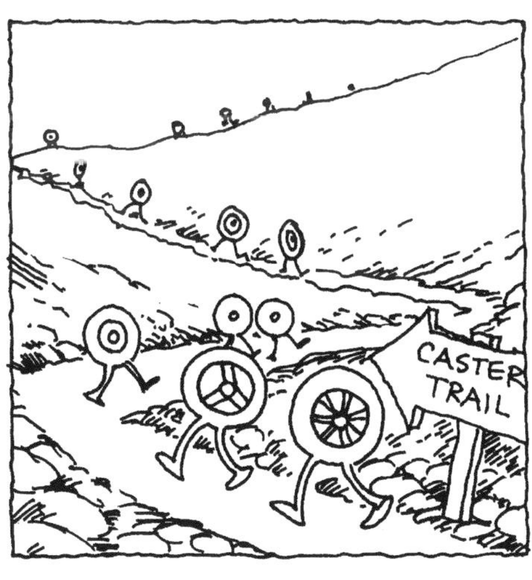

Changing the Caster Wheel Trail

It takes practice to be able to tell which direction your caster wheels are trailing. Sometimes it is hard to see their position. If you have difficulty seeing your caster wheels, practice these skills in front of a full length mirror:

- Face both caster wheels in the same direction.
- Move both caster wheels into a rearward trailing position (short wheelbase position). Do this by rolling your wheelchair forward a short distance.
- Reverse the caster wheels into the forward trailing position by rolling backward for a short distance. Lean forward and note the increased stability of your wheelchair when the caster wheels point forward.
- Make small, full rotations of the caster wheels by moving your rear wheels slightly forward, to one side, back, and then to the other side.

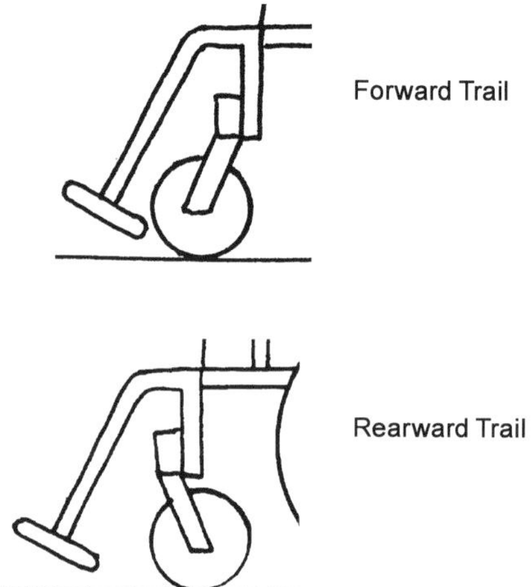

Managing Your Caster Wheels

Reverse your wheelchair to reposition your caster wheels into the forward trailing position when you want to make your wheelchair more stable in the forward direction. Some circumstances where this is recommended include:

- Transferring into and out of your wheelchair
- Moving forward on your seat cushion
- Leaning forward to reach (e.g., picking something up from the floor, reaching something on a low table or reaching something on a wall out in front of you)

Section 1.6

Relieving Pressure

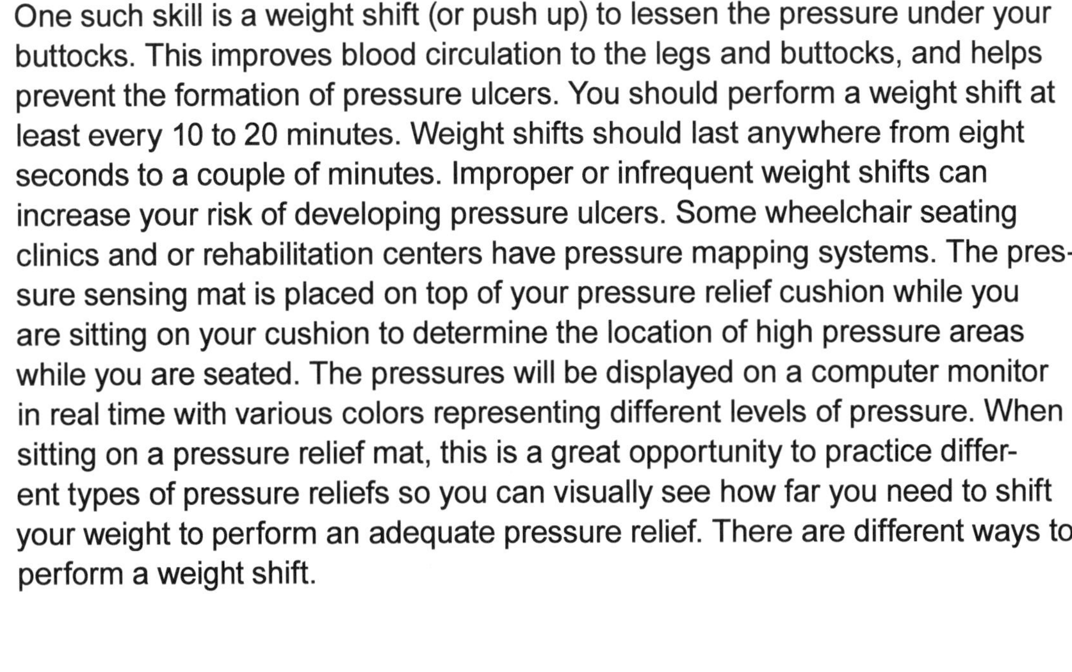

Many personal care skills take place while you are using your wheelchair. One such skill is a weight shift (or push up) to lessen the pressure under your buttocks. This improves blood circulation to the legs and buttocks, and helps prevent the formation of pressure ulcers. You should perform a weight shift at least every 10 to 20 minutes. Weight shifts should last anywhere from eight seconds to a couple of minutes. Improper or infrequent weight shifts can increase your risk of developing pressure ulcers. Some wheelchair seating clinics and or rehabilitation centers have pressure mapping systems. The pressure sensing mat is placed on top of your pressure relief cushion while you are sitting on your cushion to determine the location of high pressure areas while you are seated. The pressures will be displayed on a computer monitor in real time with various colors representing different levels of pressure. When sitting on a pressure relief mat, this is a great opportunity to practice different types of pressure reliefs so you can visually see how far you need to shift your weight to perform an adequate pressure relief. There are different ways to perform a weight shift.

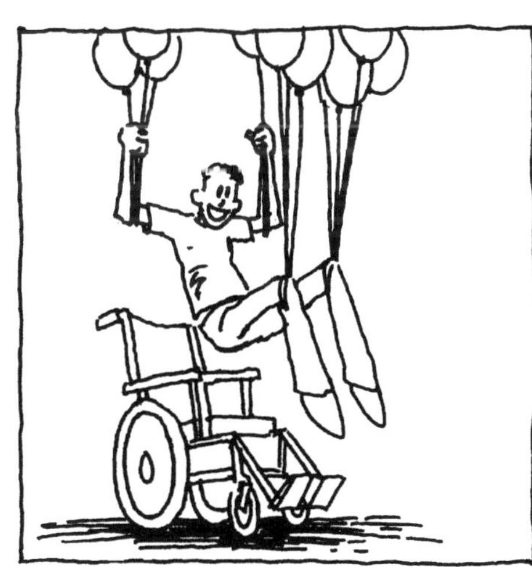

Forward Weight Shift

Resting on your body

- Put the caster wheels in the forward trailing position for stability.
- If your wheelchair has wheel locks, lock them.
- Lean your chest toward your knees, reaching down the frame of the chair.
- If you want to raise your buttocks higher, take your feet off the foot supports and position them on the floor.
- Alternatively, you can lean forward with your elbows on your knees or on the arm supports of your wheelchair.

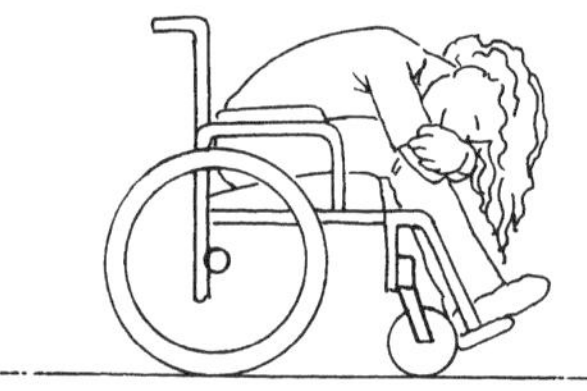

Leaning forward onto your knees helps unweight your buttocks for a pressure relief.

You can also lean on your knees to do a pressure relief weight shift.

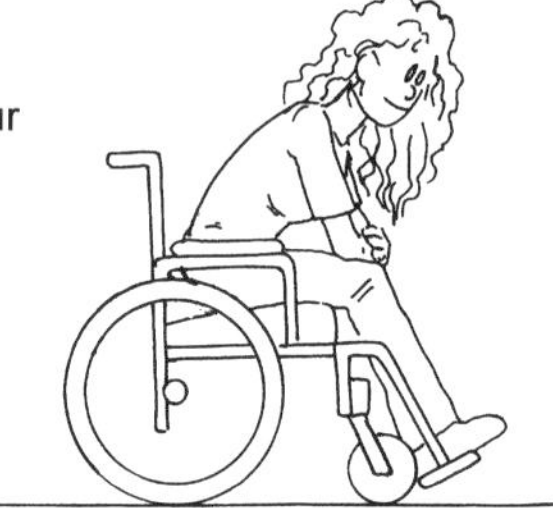

Resting on a table

- Place a pillow on a desk or table.
- Lean forward, and rest on the pillow.
- Use the desk or table to push yourself back up when finished.
- Be sure to have a spotter check that you have the weight completely off of your buttocks. Your spotter's hand should be able to fit between your buttocks and the cushion. If you do not lift your buttocks all the way off the seat, you may not be relieving the pressure enough to prevent a pressure sore from developing.

Leaning forward on a table is another way to unweight your buttocks during a pressure relief.

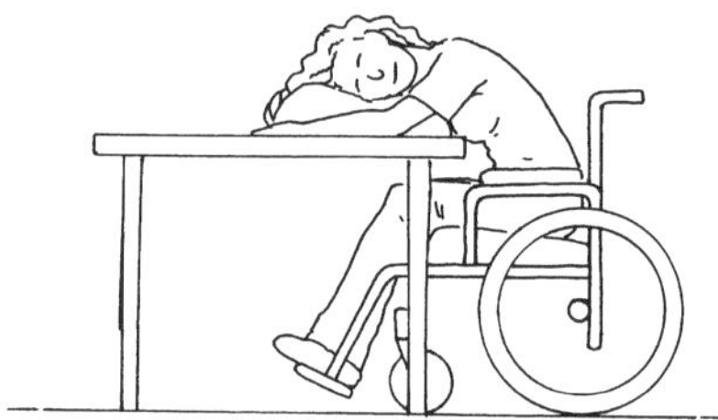

Leaning from the push handles

- Hook your arms around the push handles behind you.
- Lean forward.

Hook your arms around your push handles to avoid falling when you lean forward.

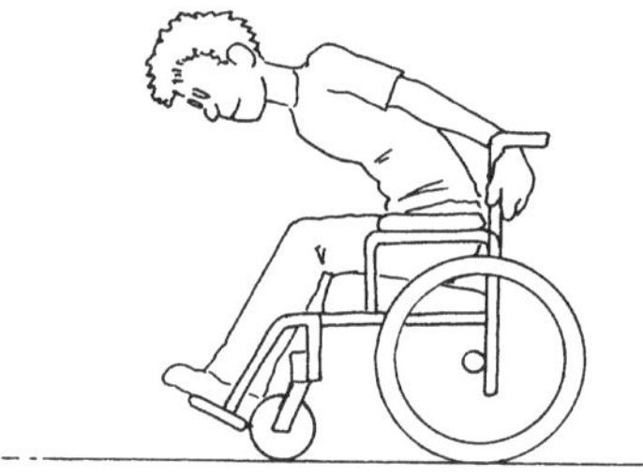

Using weight-shift loops

If you do not have good tricep strength, weight-shift loops can help you perform a forward weight shift. Weight-shift loops are looped straps attached to the back of a chair.

- Put your hands in the looped portion of your lifting straps or weight-shift loops, and lean forward.
- Pull yourself up with the weight-shift loops when ready to sit upright again.

Side-to-Side Weight Shift

Side-to-side weight shifts relieve pressure on one side of your buttocks at a time. Make sure you lean to each side so both sides of your buttocks get relief.

- Pull up parallel next to a desk, counter, wall, or bed and place the forearm closest to the object on its surface.
- Lean on the supported forearm.

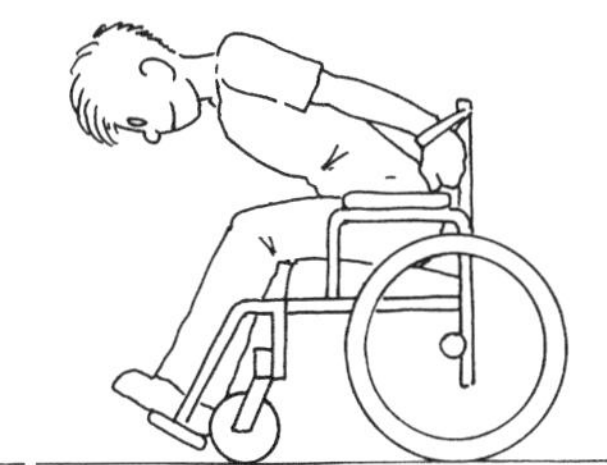

Weight-shift loops might help you perform a forward pressure relief if your triceps are weak.

- With your other hand braced on the far back support, arm support, handrim or tire, push down so you lean even further toward the desk. Be sure your buttock clears the seat.
- Turn around and do this maneuver on the other side.

Lean on a desk or other piece of furniture to help you perform a side-to-side weight shift.

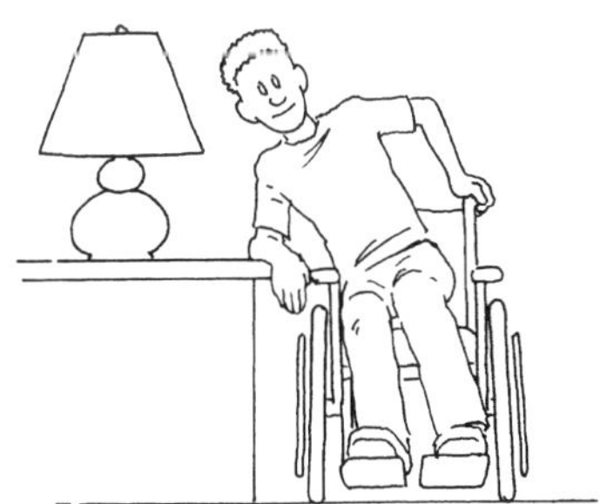

Alternatively, you can:

- Place both hands on the handrims.
- Lean to one side, alternately lifting each buttock until it clears the seat.

Push-Up Weight Shift

Warning! It is recommended that other weight shift methods be used since pushing down to lift your body weight is trying to pull your shoulder apart. This method of weight shift should only be used if your therapist feels that you have the strength in all of your rotator cuff muscles to provide your shoulders with the stability and strength necessary to perform this type of weight shift. Use other weight shift techniques whenever possible to conserve your shoulder stability for making transfers.

Tricep strength is necessary to perform this type of weight shift.

- Place your hands on the arm supports, wheels, or handrims.
- Push down through your hands until your arms are straight and your buttocks have lifted off the seat.

You can push up from arm supports, wheels, or handrims to perform a pressure relief.

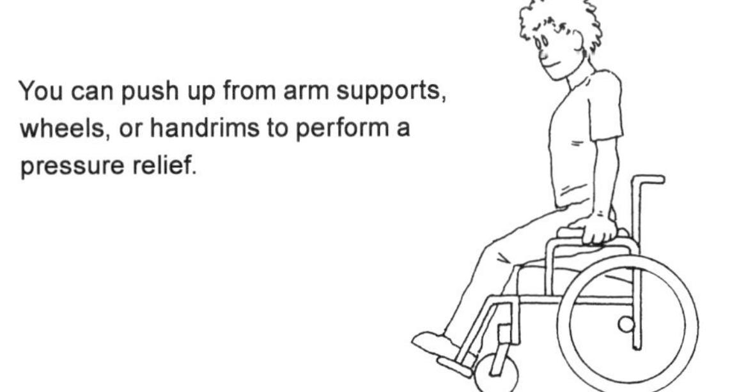

Tilting Weight Shift

Performing a tilting weight shift alone

The ability to perform a wheelie is necessary for this type of weight shift. To learn how to do this, see Section 1.9.

- Position your wheelchair directly in front of, perpendicular to, and facing away from a bed or couch.
- Pop a wheelie and lean back against the bed or couch.
- Right yourself by leaning forward while simultaneously pulling back on the wheels.
- Only lean as far forward as is necessary to right yourself.

Performing a tilting weight shift with an assistant

- Have your assistant move in front of a chair as if he/she were about to sit down on it.
- Wheel directly in front of your assistant, facing away from her/him.
- Have your assistant tip you and your wheelchair backward until he or she is sitting in the chair. The back of your wheelchair should rest on the assistant's knees or thighs.

If you are unable to perform any of the previously described weight-shifting techniques, or they do not provide sufficient relief to maintain healthy skin, have an assistant help you perform them. If you cannot do it even with someone else helping you, you should get out of your wheelchair periodically to lie on your side or stomach to relieve the pressure under your buttocks.

Section 1.7

Reaching, Bending and Lifting

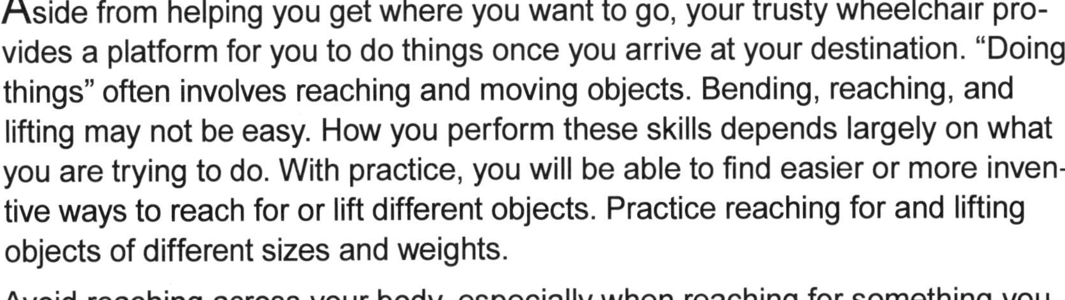

Aside from helping you get where you want to go, your trusty wheelchair provides a platform for you to do things once you arrive at your destination. "Doing things" often involves reaching and moving objects. Bending, reaching, and lifting may not be easy. How you perform these skills depends largely on what you are trying to do. With practice, you will be able to find easier or more inventive ways to reach for or lift different objects. Practice reaching for and lifting objects of different sizes and weights.

Avoid reaching across your body, especially when reaching for something you would not want to fall in your lap, such as hot coffee or a sharp knife. Twisting and lifting at the same time increases the risk of straining your back. Never try to reach for or lift objects that will exceed your capabilities. Ask for help when lifting heavy or awkward objects. Some people use trained assist dogs to pick up and retrieve objects.

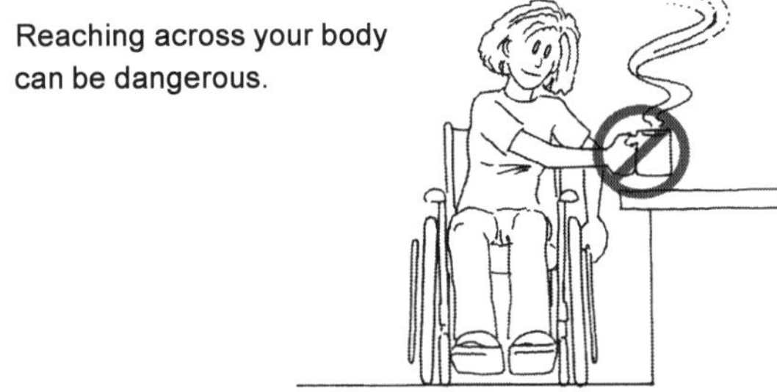

Reaching across your body can be dangerous.

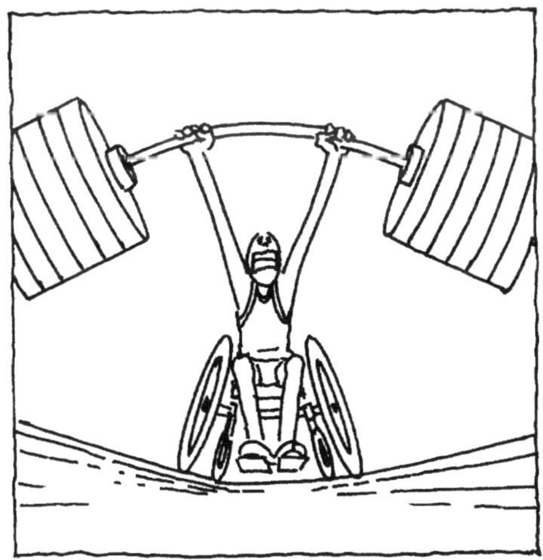

If you want to get a light object off a high store shelf, ask for assistance. If no one is available to help, use a long product in the store, such as a mop or baguette, to knock the item off the shelf. Never knock heavy or breakable objects off a shelf. Before you reach, put your caster wheels in the forward trailing position. This will lengthen your wheelbase and improve your stability. (See Section 1.5 for more information about caster wheel trail.)

Reaching Across

Reaching across your body could be dangerous. Determine the easiest and most stable way to reach and pick up objects. Sometimes, using one hand to reach and a second hand to hold onto a counter is one good way to stabilize your upper body.

Reaching Up

If you want to get a light object off a high store shelf, ask for assistance. If no one is available to help, use a long product in the store, such as a mop or baguette, to knock the item off the shelf. Never knock heavy or breakable objects off a shelf.

Reaching Forward

Before you reach, put your caster wheels in the forward trailing position. This will lengthen your wheelbase and improve your stability. (See Section 1.5 for more information about caster wheel trail.)

Reaching Sideways

If possible, pull up next to, rather than in front of, an object and reach to the side. You will most likely be more stable than if you try to reach forward or backward. You may be able to reach higher to the side than straight ahead because you will not have to reach over your wheelchair

Objects on a counter or at counter height

- Pull up next to the counter.
- Lock your wheels for added stability.
- Reach to the side for the object.
- If you need to, hold onto the opposite arm support, push handle, wheel, or counter top to help stabilize yourself.

Objects on the ground or on a low shelf

- Pull up so the object is to the side of your wheelchair.
- Rotate your front caster wheels so they point toward the direction you are reaching.
- Hook your arm around the push handle or grab the back post or wheel on your wheelchair's side opposite the object. Holding onto the wheel affords more stability when reaching sideways to pick something up off the floor.
- Lean down to pick up the object with your free arm.
- When you have grasped the object, pull yourself up with the arm around the push handle or back of your wheelchair.

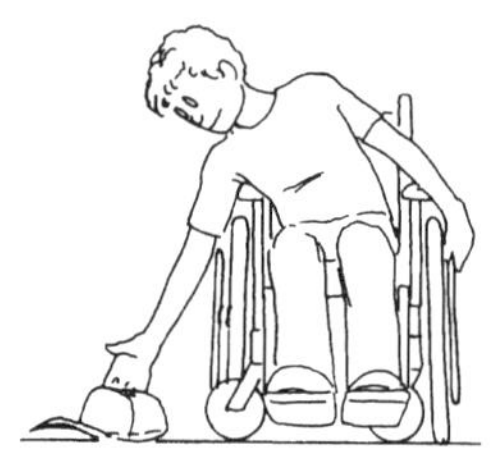

Holding onto the wheel affords more stability when picking up something off the floor sideways.

How a spotter can help

- Stand to the side of the wheelchair user opposite the object that the wheelchair user is lifting.
- Be ready to keep the wheelchair user from falling forward out of their wheelchair.
- Be ready to keep their wheelchair from tipping. It may be helpful to put your foot on the bottom of the wheel rim on the side you are on.

Helpful Hint

Avoid reaching for objects with your weaker hand. Instead, turn around and use your stronger hand to grasp and lift.

Reaching Forward

The ability to reach forward is useful to tie your shoes, pick up objects from the floor, or to empty a leg bag. You can also use your foot supports, feet, and/or knees to help lift the object into your lap in stages.

Smaller and/or lighter objects

Basic forward reach

- Make sure your caster wheels are in the forward trailing position.
- Lean forward with one forearm laid across your knees, or firmly grab your wheelchair frame in front of the seat for support, and reach forward with the other hand.
- Lift the object onto your feet or foot support.
- Push your free forearm against your knees or push down on your wheelchair frame with your hand to raise yourself up, pulling the object into your lap at the same time.

Place your forearm across your legs for more trunk support.

Braced forward reach

- Make sure your caster wheels are in the forward trailing position.
- Bend forward, resting your chest on your knees.
- Reach forward with one hand, and lift the object onto your feet or foot support.
- Hook the other arm around the push handle or back of your wheelchair, and pull yourself up.
- Leaning forward slightly, grab the object and lift it onto your lap.

Diagonal forward reach

- Make sure your caster wheels are in the forward trailing position.
- Hook an arm around the back of your wheelchair.
- Bend forward and rest on your knee, bracing yourself with the arm hooked around the push handle or wheelchair back.
- Reach forward with your free hand and lift the object onto your feet and then into your lap.
- Pull yourself upright using the arm you have hooked around the push handle or back of your wheelchair.

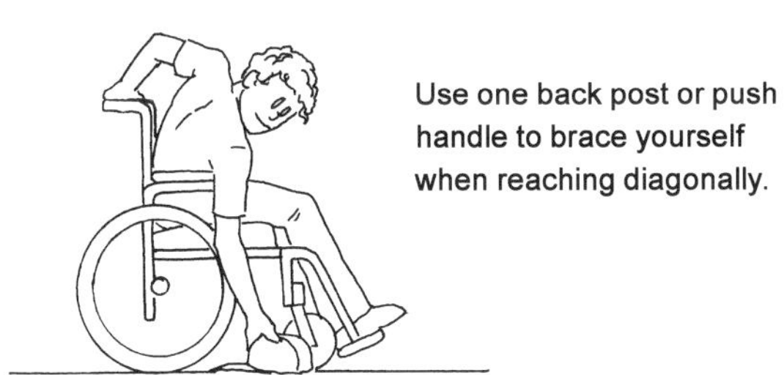

Use one back post or push handle to brace yourself when reaching diagonally.

Helpful Hint

There are many adaptive devices available to help you reach for objects. They include, but are not limited to:

- canes
- dressing sticks
- reachers
- hangers
- button hook devices
- double-stick tape on rulers
- magnet on a stick
- tongs (barbecue and scissor types)

Larger and/or heavier objects

- Make sure your caster wheels are in the forward trailing position.
- Bend forward and rest your chest on your knees.
- Grasping the object, lift it with both hands onto your feet.
- While the object is resting on your feet, pull yourself upright by pushing on your knees or hooking your arm around the push handle or back of the chair.
- Lean forward slightly to grasp the object.
- Lift the object onto your knees or lap.

How the spotter can help

- Be sure the caster wheels are in a forward trailing position.
- Stand to the side of the wheelchair user opposite the object the wheelchair user is picking up.
- Be ready to keep the user from falling and their wheelchair from tipping forward or to the side.

Section 1.8

Propelling Your Wheelchair

While propelling a wheelchair forward and backward might seem intuitive, performing these actions incorrectly can cause fatigue, waste energy, and lead to hand, wrist, and shoulder strain. You can propel your wheelchair by grasping the handrims, the tires, or the handrims and tires simultaneously. Many people use handrims, while others remove them because they want a narrower wheelchair or prefer to directly grasp the tires. Your hands might getter dirtier if you propel using the tires instead of the handrims unless you wear gloves.

There are different styles of handrims that might make it easier for you to propel your wheelchair. (See Section 1.2 under the Wheels subsection for more information). You can also wrap rubber tubing around the handrims to make them easier to grip. Handrims coated with grip enhancing rubber or plastic are also available. Gloves can help improve your grip, prevent blisters and calluses from developing, and can shield your hands from tire grime. Remember that when gloves get wet, they may cause your hands to slip as well. Leather gloves without fingertips are sold by sailing equipment suppliers, gloves with padded palms are available in bicycle shops or sporting good stores, and cotton gardening gloves with rubber grips can be found in nurseries and home improvement stores.

Wheel locks may get in your way during propulsion. Some experienced wheelchair users remove or turn them upside down to get them out of the way. Swing away wheel locks are also available that move completely out of the way when not in use.

In general, shorter push strokes provide better control, while longer push strokes provide more push, so you might want to use short strokes in small, tight environments and longer strokes in more open areas. Longer strokes are usually more efficient and may make you less tired.

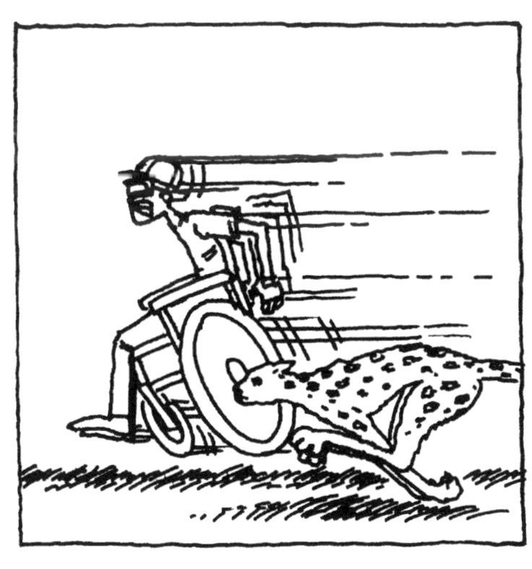

Hand Positioning

Putting your hands at the right places will help you get the most push with the least effort. To learn proper hand positioning, think of your right rear wheel as the face of a clock. Twelve o'clock is the top center of the wheel, two o'clock is in front of you and eleven o'clock is behind you.

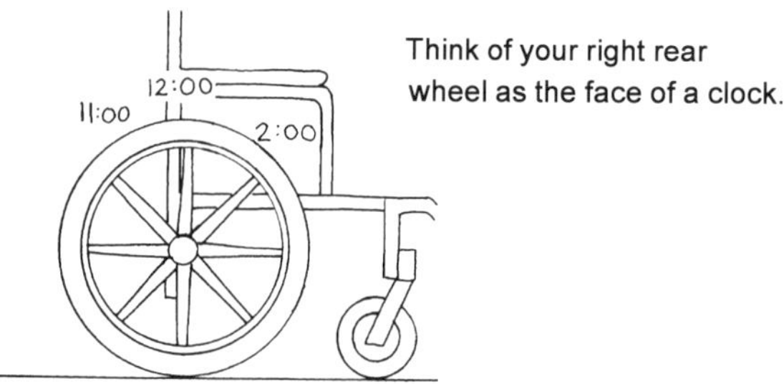

Think of your right rear wheel as the face of a clock.

Grasp the handrims with your fingers. Avoid wrapping your thumbs around the handrims. Instead, position your thumbs along the inside top surface of the handrims and point them forward.

If you do not have the hand function required to grasp the handrims, use the heels of your hands to push the wheels forward. This method is known as the friction technique.

Some ergonomic handrims, like the Flexrims™, are designed for the users to push using just the heel of their hand without the requirement to squeeze or grip the handrim.

Push with the heels of your hands if you cannot wrap your fingers around the handrims.

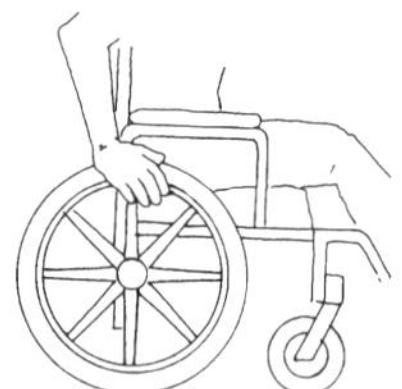

Basic Propulsion Stroke

How far back you reach to grasp your handrims and/or tires depends on your strength, flexibility, and the speed you are trying to maintain. Generally, long and even strokes conserve the most energy and will cause less strain on your shoulders. The following is a basic technique for propelling your wheelchair:

- Reach your hands behind you and grasp the handrims and/or tires at 11:00 or 12:00.
- Propel forward to 2:00 and release.
- Let your hands drop slightly and loop in a circular manner back to the hand rim.
- Reach behind to 11:00 or 12:00 again, and repeat the maneuver.

This method helps keep your strokes smooth and even, and will reduce the strain on your shoulders. A "bigger" motion will cause more shoulder strain. Try to be consistent in your stroke length to propel more efficiently. If you cannot reach 2:00 and 11:00 or 12:00, reassess your sitting position. An improperly adjusted wheelchair is difficult to propel. You may be able to lower your seat or raise your rear wheels so you can reach the wheels better. If you are still unable to reach back to 11:00, try 12:00 to 2:00 or even 12:00 to 1:00. A quick check for proper wheel position relative to your seat is the "index finger to wheel axle test". While sitting comfortably against the backrest, drop your hands to either side. The tip of your index finger should rest close to the middle of the wheel axle.

It is important that following a push, you "recover" below the rim. When you are bringing your arm back from the 2:00 position to the 11:00 position, you should do it below, not above, the handrim of the chair.

(See Section 1.2 for more information about setting up your wheelchair.)

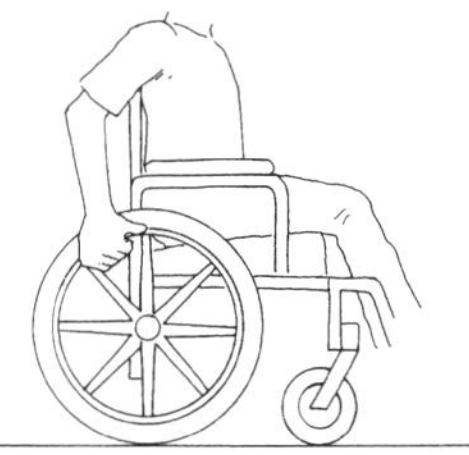

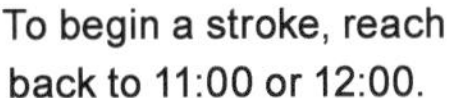

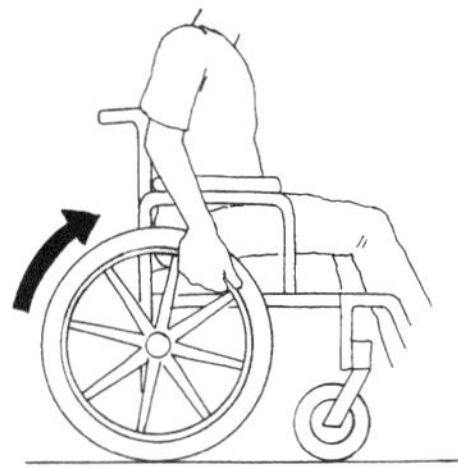

To begin a stroke, reach back to 11:00 or 12:00.

Push forward to 2:00, then reach back to 11:00 or 12:00, and push again.

Hand-to-Hand (Left-to-Right) Propulsion

Pushing hand to hand is a good way to maintain your forward momentum up a ramp or across a rough surface. This method gives a rougher ride, but can help you maintain momentum. When using the techniques described above, there is a pause every time your hands reach back to take another stroke. When you push hand to hand, there is no pause in forward momentum between strokes.

- If you can, lean forward a little bit to maintain your balance.
- With your left hand, reach back to the 11:00 or 12:00 position, as before, and grab the handrim and/or tire. As you push forward with your left hand, reach back with your right hand and grab the 11:00 or 12:00 position on the right handrim and/or tire.
- As you release your left hand, push forward with your right.
- As you are pushing with your right hand, be sure that your left hand is reaching back and gripping the left handrim and/or tire.
- Continue alternating hands to propel your wheelchair. On a slope this type of propulsion may cause your wheelchair to weave a lot and this can be uncomfortable or even dangerous, so use wisdom as to when to use this method, and caution, when you do.

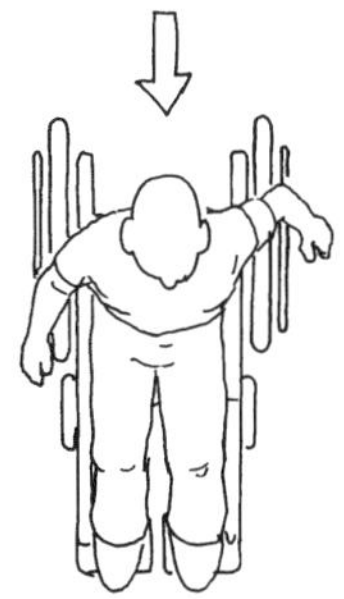

Use the hand-to-hand technique to push with one hand, maintaining forward momentum.

Propelling Backward

Propelling your wheelchair backward is useful for basic maneuvering and is necessary to perform advanced maneuvers such as climbing curbs and stairs.

- Look behind you to make sure the path is clear.
- Begin by reaching your hands in front of you to about the 2:00 position on the wheel and grab the tires and/or handrims.
- Pull backward to the 11:00 or 12:00 position and release.
- Reach forward and repeat the maneuver.

Turning Your Wheelchair

Turning in a wheelchair is accomplished by making the left and right rear wheels turn at different speeds. (NOTE: The directions given here are for left turns only. By simply changing the instruction to the opposite hands, you will attain the same right turns.)

Wide left turn

- Hold the left handrim and/or tire at the top position.
- Push forward on the right handrim and/or tire.
- Your wheelchair will turn to the left.

The further behind and forward you reach with your right hand the more you will turn with one push. You can make an even wider turn by just slowing the left handrim from rolling, rather than stopping it completely. This technique is often used when you are moving at a steady pace and need to turn just a little bit (see moving left turn below).

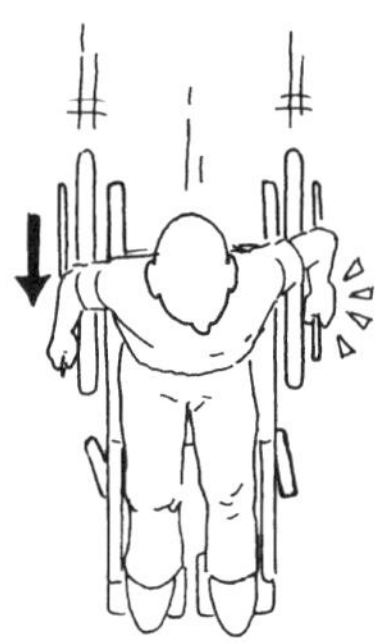

Push with one hand and hold with the other hand to make a wide turn.

Sharp left turn

- Reach forward with your left hand and grab the left handrim and/or tire at 2:00.
- At the same time, reach behind you with your right hand and grab the right handrim and/or tire at 11:00 or 12:00.
- Simultaneously pull back with your left hand and push forward with your right hand.
- Your wheelchair will turn sharply to the left.
- The farther forward and behind you reach, the more you will turn with one push.
- Pull back on one wheel and push forward on the other to make a sharp turn.

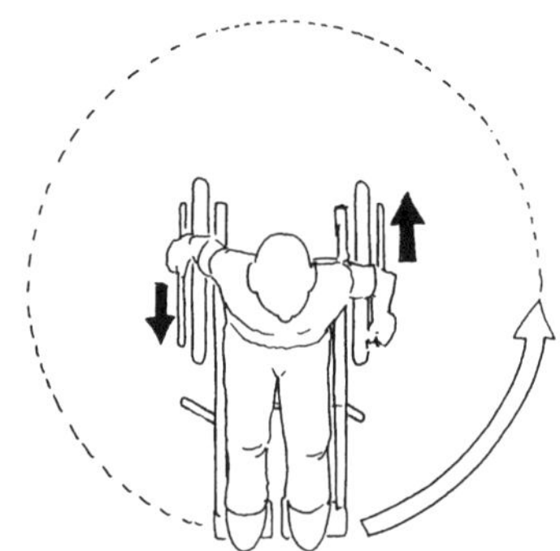

Pull back on one wheel and push forward on the other to make a sharp turn.

Moving left turn

- Propel your wheelchair forward.
- When you are ready to turn, brake by pressing your left hand flat against the handrim or tire while continuing to propel with the right hand.
- Your wheelchair will turn to the left.

The severity of the turn can be controlled by how much drag you apply to the handrim. The more you stop the left wheel, the sharper you will turn.

Section 1.9

Wheelies

The wheelie is an important basic skill that can dramatically expand your mobility options. Among other things, popping a wheelie makes it easier to go up and down curbs, descend ramps and other slopes, and smooth the ride over doorsills, bumps and small obstacles. A wheelie can even help you impress friends with dance floor spins!

Chair setup significantly affects wheelie technique. Moving the rear wheels forward increases the chair's tip ability and makes it easier to pop a wheelie. Set up your wheelchair so it is easy, but not too easy, to pop a wheelie. This will make your wheelchair reasonably stable while retaining maneuverability. (See Section 1.2 for more information about adjusting your wheelchair). Your body positioning will also affect your wheelchair's stability. The farther forward your weight is relative to the rear axle, the less tippy your wheelchair will be. The tippier the chair setup, the less weight shifting you will have to do to pop a wheelie. It should be noted that it is easier to initially learn to balance in a wheelie on a soft surface such as on a padded plush carpet.

Before you attempt to learn wheelies, you should be able to propel both forward and backward using the wheels or handrims. When performing wheelies, relax your body and sit all the way back in your wheelchair seat. Muscle tension and upper-body movements dramatically affect your balance point. With practice, you will be able to control your balance with subtle upper body movements.

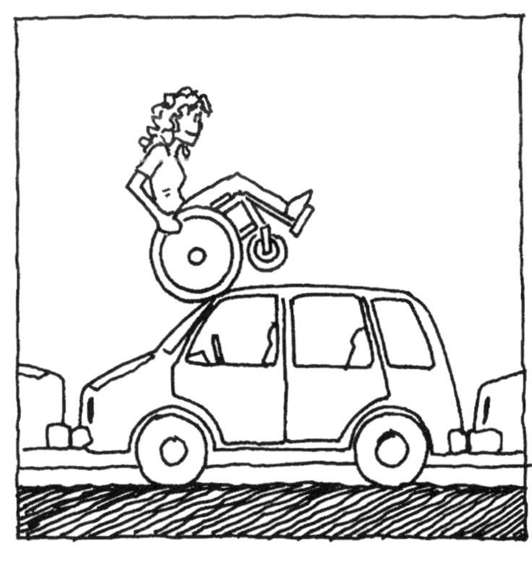

Remember that learning wheelies may not be realistic for everyone. Performing the techniques in this section may expose you, and any assistants helping you, to physical strain and or serious injury. When learning wheelies, the use of a spotter with a spotting strap is highly recommended.

NOTE: Before practicing wheelies, read the warning on page vi to learn the risks involved in learning wheelie skills. Remember that falling is an unacceptable option for some wheelchair users, and may result in severe injury or death. It is extremely important to learn wheelies with a physical or occupational therapist or a RESNA certified Assistive Technology Professional (ATP) with experience in wheelchair training.

Use of a Spotter Strap

During maneuvers where you will be learning to do a wheelie or there is a risk of tipping to the rear, the use of a simple webbing strap that is attached underneath the back of your wheelchair and held by your spotter or assistant following behind you is highly encouraged for the safety of both you and your spotter or assistant. The benefits of a spotter or spotting strap as outlined by the Wheelchair Skills Program developed at Dalhousie University in Halifax, NS, in Canada, are the following:

- Reduces the likelihood of injury due to rear-tipping accidents.
- Reduces the likelihood of injury due to the wheelchair "running away" on downhill grades.
- Provides confidence when learning new skills or attempting to use the wheelchair in challenging environments.
- Allows a spotter to stand farther away from the wheelchair than would be appropriate without the spotter strap.
- Eliminates the need for the spotter to bend forward to catch a tipping wheelchair.
- Allows effective spotting even for wheelchairs without push handles or lifting straps.

A spotter strap can be made by tying or sewing a loop at each end of a webbing strap or piece of rope. It is recommended to attach a spotter strap near the midline of the wheelchair to avoid inducing lateral instabilities during its use. For a wheelchair with a cross-brace that permits the wheelchair to be folded, connect the spotter strap around the cross brace. For a rigid-frame wheelchair with a horizontal frame member, connect the spotter strap tightly around the center of the horizontal frame member. Be sure to run the spotter strap up between the back support of the wheelchair and any backpack that the user might be used to wearing on the back of the wheelchair. Practice using the spotter strap with another assistant or spotter to learn to catch a tipping wheelchair as early as possible to minimize the forces involved. For more in-depth instructions or for instructions on making, purchasing or using spotter straps, contact the Wheelchair Skills Program at Dalhousie University (www.wheelchairskillsprogram.ca).

Partial Wheelies

Popping your caster wheels off the ground for a short period of time is called a partial wheelie, "popping your caster wheels up," or "popping up." Use this technique to go over thresholds, curbs, and other small obstacles. Popping a partial wheelie requires lifting the front caster wheels from the ground when popping a full wheelie may not be necessary. Start practicing partial wheelies on smooth, flat surfaces. Look for irregularities in the surface, which could cause you to lose your balance. As you increase your proficiency at popping partial wheelies, practice popping them as you cross cracks in the sidewalk. This will help you practice lining up your wheelchair and will improve your timing. Once you can do this, try it over small obstacles like doorsills.

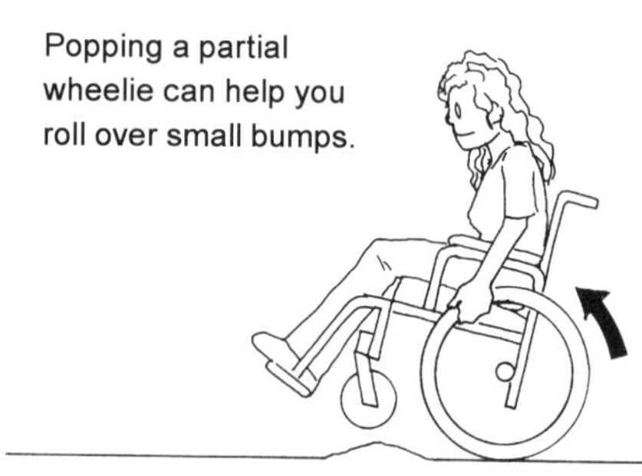

Popping a partial wheelie can help you roll over small bumps.

Popping a partial wheelie

- Back away slightly from the transition you wish to cross.
- Push forward quickly as you shift your head and shoulders forward slightly. This will momentarily lift the front caster wheels off the ground to cross the transition.

How a spotter can help

- Attach a spotter strap to the wheelchair so you can prevent the wheelchair user from falling over backwards during the learning process.
- Stand behind the wheelchair user while holding the spotter strap in one hand so you are ready to prevent a rearward tip. Try not to influence the balance of the wheelchair user.
- Move in the same direction and at the same pace as the wheelchair user.
- As the wheelchair user comes down to the ground, keep one hand on the rider's shoulder to keep him/her from falling forward.

Balance Point

The balance point is reached when you can tip back to balance on the two large rear wheels, with your front caster wheels in the air. You have to be able to find and maintain your balance point in order to maintain a wheelie.

Finding your balance point

- Have your spotter attach a spotter strap to the wheelchair to prevent you from falling over backwards during the learning process.
- Have your spotter tip your wheelchair back into a balanced wheelie by pushing down on the push handles, back posts, and/or anti-tip device. Anti-tip devices may have to be removed or flipped up before your wheelchair will tip back into a wheelie.
- To feel how your seat moves in relation to your wheels, hold your wheels still as you are being tipped back.
- Have the spotter hold your wheelchair in the wheelie position so you both become familiar with how to find your balance point, which is often farther back than expected.

A spotter can tip your wheelchair into a wheelie to help you find your balance point.

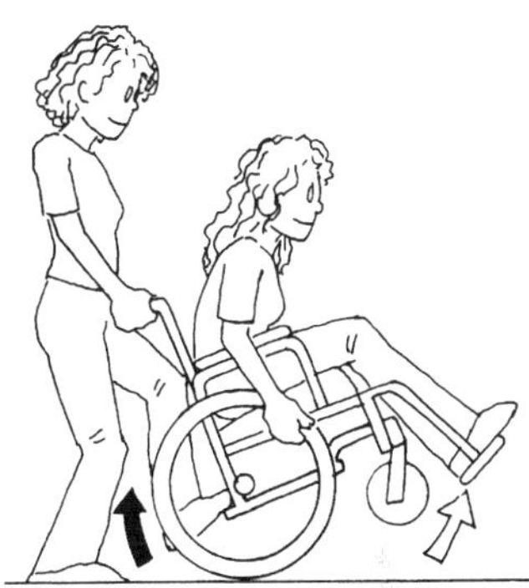

- When you start feeling comfortable with your balance point, try to hold yourself in that position as your spotter releases his or her grip on the push handle or back support. Your spotter's hand should hold the handle or pull strap very loosely to avoid affecting your balance. The spotter should always hold onto the spotter strap with their other hand.
- You will probably have to make slight adjustments by rolling your wheels forward and back, and leaning forward and back to keep your balance. Push forward on your wheels to bring the front end up. Pull backward on your wheels to bring the front end down.

Wheelies

Actually popping a wheelie requires you to lift your caster wheels off the ground far enough for you to reach your balance point. Popping a wheelie when rolling backward or from a stationary position takes less strength and timing than trying to pop one while rolling forward.

When first learning to do a wheelie, roll your wheelchair backward to create some backward momentum before pushing forward into the wheelie.

At first, practice wheelies on soft surfaces such as carpet or grass which will not allow the rear wheels to move as quickly as on a hard surface. In addition, softer surfaces will help cushion any falls. As your technique improves, you can practice on hard, smooth surfaces. Be sure to look for and avoid surface irregularities, bumps or cracks which can cause your wheelchair to tip over. When learning wheelie skills, always enlist the help of a spotter.

How a spotter can help with all wheelie skills

- Attach a spotter strap to the wheelchair so you can prevent the wheelchair user from falling over backwards during the learning process.
- Position yourself behind the wheelchair user with one hand holding onto a spotter strap. Try not to influence the balance of the wheelchair user.
- Move at the same pace as the wheelchair user.
- Prevent the wheelchair user from tipping too far backward.
- Initially you can assist the wheelchair user to balance using the hand that is not holding the spotter strap to hold the push handle or back support of the wheelchair.

Popping a Wheelie

- Pull on the handrims to roll backward a short distance.
- While rolling backwards, push forward somewhat aggressively on the handrims as you shift your head and shoulders forward slightly.
- Most people are initially more comfortable when they lean their head and shoulders forward slightly, however with experience, you will find that leaning back in your chair will require the wheelchair to tip back less to balance.
- When you reach the balance point, your hands will be forward at about the 1:00 position on the handrim.
- If you find yourself tipping forward, push forward on the handrims and/or lean back to regain your balance point.
- If you find yourself tipping backward, pull back on the handrims and/or lean forward to regain your balance point.
- Pull back on the handrims to bring your wheelchair back down onto all four wheels.
- If you feel like you are falling over backwards, pull back aggressively on the handrims to bring your wheelchair back down onto all four wheels.
- Practice stationary wheelies until you can release your hands to move back and forth slightly, re-gripping the handrims as needed to stay balanced in a wheelie.

Popping a wheelie

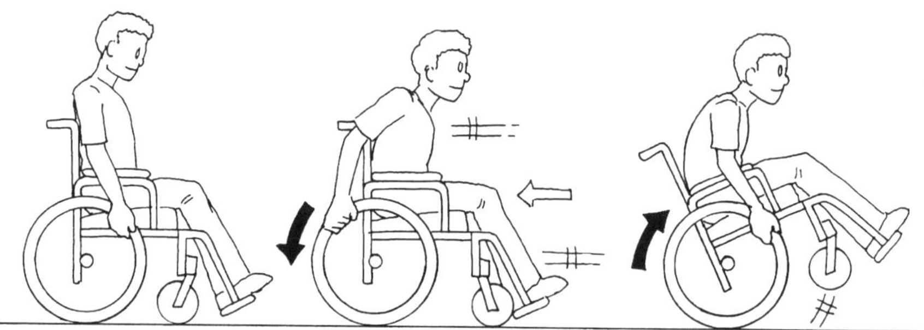

1. Roll backward.
2. Grab the handrims.
3. Rapidly push forward on the handrims as you shift your head and shoulders forward slightly.

Wheelies from Motion

Popping a wheelie while in motion allows you to climb up curbs or over obstacles quickly and easily using momentum. Popping a wheelie while rolling forward is a little more difficult than popping a wheelie when rolling backward or from a standstill.

Rolling forward wheelies

- Roll your wheelchair forward, slowly at first.
- When ready to pop the wheelie, reach back and grasp the handrims and/or wheels behind you. Push forward quickly and lightly shift your weight backward at the same time.
- When you reach the balance point, you will want your hands centered on top of the wheels so you can continue to propel forward in a wheelie.
- Once you have mastered popping a wheelie while moving slowly, try it at faster speeds.

Moving in a Wheelie

Once you can maintain a stationary wheelie easily, practice rolling forward and backward in the wheelie position. Learning to move forward and backward in a wheelie position can be difficult, frightening, or uncomfortable because you have to let yourself fall slightly forward or backward.

Moving forward in a wheelie

To move forward in a wheelie, you must let yourself tip slightly forward. As you begin to tip forward, push forward gently on the handrims to maintain your balance. Repeating this movement will move you forward across the floor in a wheelie.

Repeat the maneuver, making your way slowly across the floor. You may move awkwardly at first, but with practice you will get faster and the movement will be smoother and require less effort.

If you start tipping too far forward, push forward on the handrims and lean back to regain your balance point. If you start tipping backward, pull back on the handrims and lean forward to regain your balance point.

As you become more comfortable with this maneuver, try rolling forward in a wheelie over longer distances.

Moving backward in a wheelie

Moving backward in a wheelie is a similar maneuver. You have to let yourself tip slightly backward, then pull back on your handrims to maintain your balance.

- Pop a wheelie.
- Allow yourself to tip slightly backward, then pull back on the handrims to regain your balance.
- Repeat this maneuver, slowly making your way across the floor. At first you will move awkwardly, but your wheelies will get faster and smoother with practice.
- If you find yourself tipping too far backward, pull back on the handrims and lean forward to regain your balance.
- If you feel like you are falling over backwards, pull back aggressively on the handrims to bring your wheelchair back down onto all four wheels.
- As you become more comfortable with this maneuver, try rolling backwards for longer distances.

Staying in wheelie position

To turn your wheelchair in the wheelie position, you must let go of the wheels for short periods of time. Therefore, the first step toward learning to turn in a wheelie is learning to hold yourself in the wheelie position with one hand.

- Pop a wheelie.
- Lift one hand off the handrim and try to keep your balance with the other hand.
- Alternate between hands until you are comfortable balancing in a wheelie using either hand.

Pivoting in a wheelie

- Pop a wheelie.
- While maintaining the wheelie position, pull with your left hand, and push with your right.
- Your wheelchair will rotate to the left.

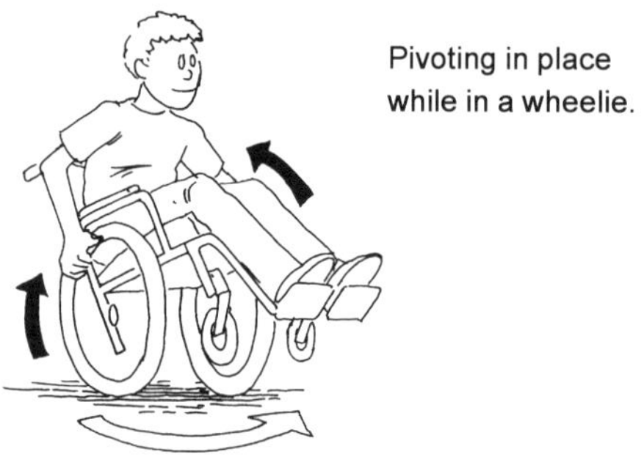

Pivoting in place while in a wheelie.

Moving wheelie turn

- Pop a wheelie and propel your wheelchair forward.
- While maintaining the wheelie position, press your left hand flat against the handrim or tire to slow or stop it from rolling while continuing to propel with your right hand.
- Your wheelchair will turn to the left.
- Pull back on the left handrim to make a sharper turn.

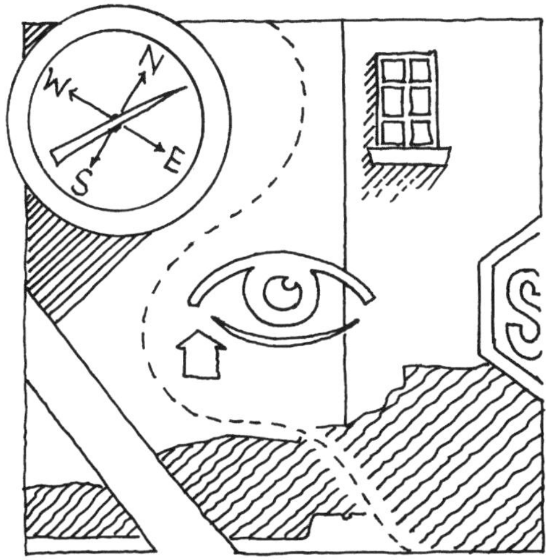

Chapter 2

Navigation Skills

As just about everyone since Columbus knows, the world is not flat, nor is it uniformly smooth, level, firm, stable, or slip resistant, despite changes brought by the Americans with Disabilities Act. There are still stairs to climb, doors to open and close, and lawns to cross. Your wheelchair can help you access these terrain types once you learn the navigation skills in this chapter. You already have a great start if you mastered wheelies.

Before practicing the maneuvers in this section, read the warning on page vi to learn about the risks involved in performing wheelchair skills. Many of the skills in this section require a lot of experience and really good balance. Most people fall at some point while performing these techniques. Section 3.1 contains information on how to fall safely. It is important to practice falling safely before you try these skills. Remember that falling is an unacceptable option for some wheelchair users and falling may result in severe injury or death.

Sections in This Chapter

Section 2.1

Smooth Surfaces

The surfaces you cross greatly affect your wheelchair's ride and performance. The easiest type of surface to cross is smooth, level, firm, stable, and slip resistant. These surfaces are usually found in public buildings such as schools, offices, and shopping malls, and are often made of wood, linoleum, or concrete.

If you notice your wheelchair pulling to one side or performing oddly when rolling over such an ideal surface, it is probably due to a problem with your wheelchair. This might stem from having more camber set in one wheel than the other, from a wheel or wheels that toe in or out, or from tires with unequal air pressure.

Your wheels and tires will also affect your wheelchair's performance. Hard, narrow tires are best on smooth surfaces. If you plan to use your wheelchair on a variety of surfaces, select tires and wheels that offer better traction. (See Section 1.2 for more information on how tires affect wheelchair performance.) If the surface is truly smooth, firm, stable, and slip resistant, crossing it is a matter of simple propulsion. (See Section 1.8 for more information about propelling your wheelchair.) Nevertheless, you should still watch for:

- changes in surface type such as from wood to linoleum
- objects such as tacks or pens on the floor
- wet or sticky patches such as spilled juice or water

The more uneven the terrain, the rougher the ride you will experience. Seams between surfaces such as wood flooring and carpet can require special preparation and maneuvering to cross. Even on smooth surfaces, you should watch for cracks, grooves, and pits that can catch your caster wheels.

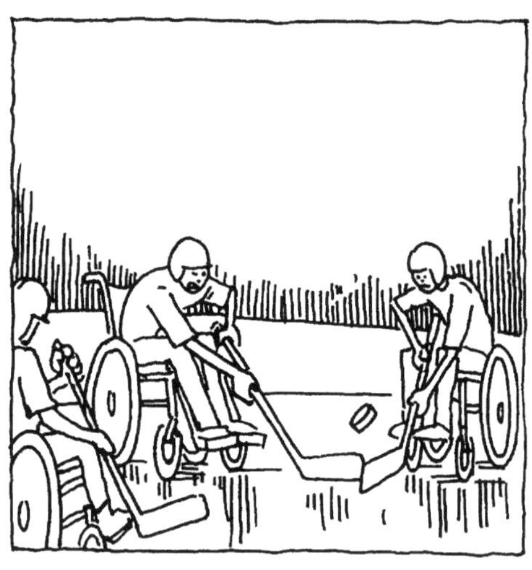

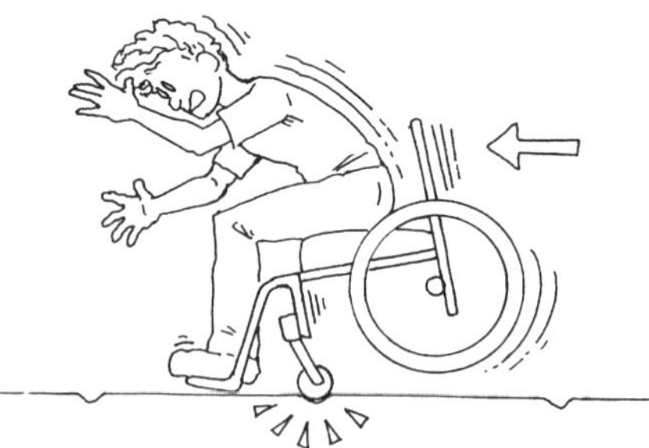

Even on smooth surfaces, you should watch for cracks, grooves, and pits that can catch your casters.

Section 2.2

Thresholds and Obstacles

A threshold is the raised bump in a doorway that prevents water and air drafts from leaking into a room. Usually made of wood or metal, thresholds vary in height and present obstacles to many wheelchair users. It can be difficult to gather enough forward momentum to roll over thresholds and other obstacles if there is little runway room or the surface is rough. Wheelchairs with large front caster wheels can climb over thresholds and obstacles more easily than smaller caster wheels, which may catch on objects, such as thresholds, and pitch you forward in the path of travel. (See Section 1.2 for more information about wheels and tires.)

Before learning how to cross thresholds and negotiate obstacles, you should be able to propel forward and backward independently. Minimal trunk control and upper extremity strength are needed to cross very low thresholds and obstacles. Trunk control and arm strength become more important as obstacles get bigger.

Make sure your foot supports are positioned properly before practicing the maneuvers in this section. A low foot support can catch on thresholds, curb ramps, and other obstacles and cause your wheelchair to tip forward. Set your foot supports at least two inches off the ground. If this position causes your knees to wobble, raise your seat or use a thicker cushion. Consider using foot supports with plastic skid plates or wheels to avoid running aground on curb ramps or other obstacles. If you do not have enough foot support clearance to roll over the obstacle, you will need to pop a partial wheelie over it or ask someone for assistance. Anti-tip devices can be adjusted high enough for you to pop the caster wheels over obstacles. If a spotter is helping you negotiate thresholds and obstacles, use a spotter strap as described and explained in Section 1.9 Wheelies.

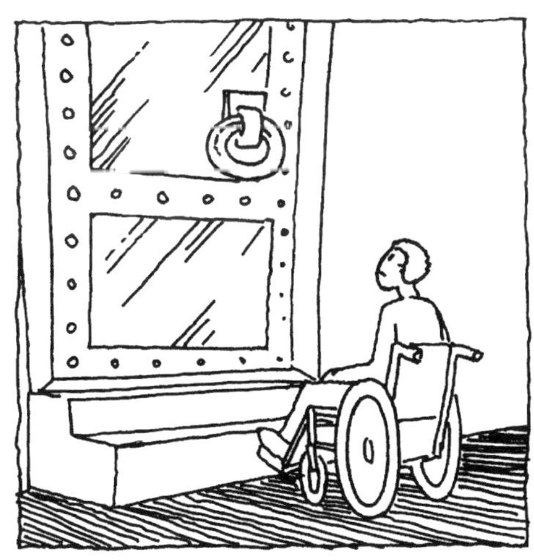

Footplate wheels can help you travel over obstacles and across slope transitions more smoothly.

Take safety precautions when learning to cross thresholds and obstacles. If you have poor trunk balance, try using a chest strap for more support. Always have a spotter nearby to catch you in case you start falling while practicing. Moving over a threshold or obstacle essentially requires two crossings: one to move the front caster wheels over and the other to bring the rear wheels over.

Basic Threshold or Obstacle Crossing

- Roll your wheelchair forward until the front caster wheels rest against the threshold or obstacle.
- Lean backward slightly and push forward on the handrims, moving the caster wheels up and over the threshold or obstacle. Some people prefer to ease the caster wheels over the obstacle one at a time. (See Section 1.9 on how to pop your front caster wheels off the ground.)
- Lean forward and push forward strongly to maneuver the rear wheels over the threshold or obstacle. Leaning forward brings your weight forward and makes it easier to push the rear wheels over an obstacle.

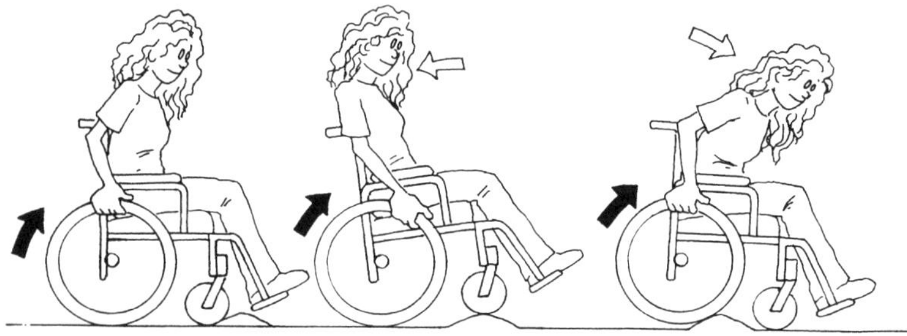

1. Roll your caster wheels up to meet the threshold.
2. Lean back and pop your front caster wheels up and over the threshold.
3. Lean forward to make rolling your rear wheels over the threshold easier.

Using a Door Frame

- Roll your wheelchair forward until the front caster wheels rest against the threshold.
- Lean backward slightly and push forward on the handrims, moving the caster wheels up and over the threshold. (See Section 1.9 on how to pop a partial wheelie to get your front caster wheels off the ground.)
- Making sure the door will not close on your fingers, reach through the doorway and grasp the far side of the door-frame with both hands.
- Pull yourself through the doorway until your rear wheels have crossed the threshold.

1. After popping your caster wheels over the threshold, reach through the doorway and grasp the other side of the door frame.

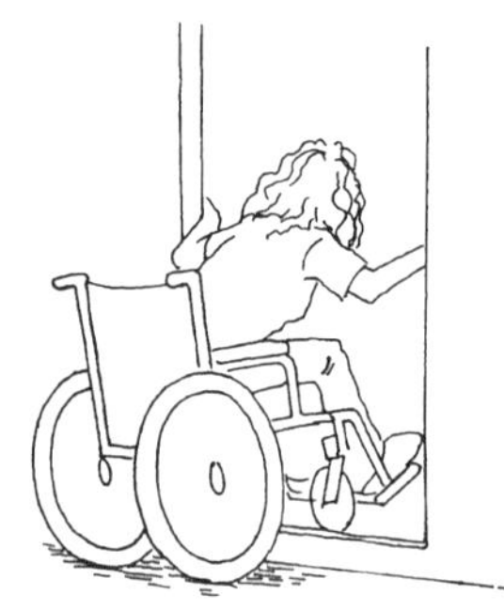

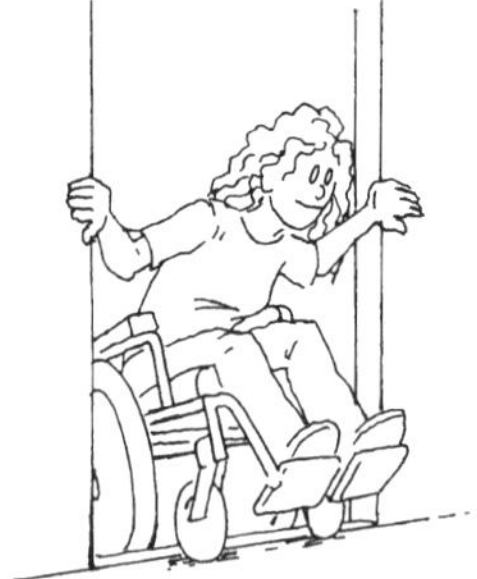

2. Pull yourself through the doorway until your rear wheels cross the threshold.

How a spotter can help

- Stand behind the wheelchair with one hand close to the push handles or near the back support posts with the pull straps and the other hand positioned over one of the rider's shoulders. In this position you can prevent the wheelchair from tipping too far back or the rider from falling forward.
- Place one foot in front of the other in a wide stance and use your forward thigh to push forward against the back of the wheelchair if needed.
- Be ready to catch the rider at the shoulders if she or he loses trunk stability in the forward direction.

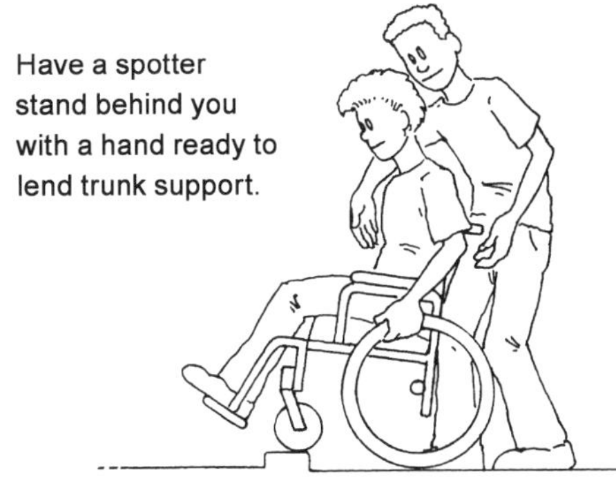
Have a spotter stand behind you with a hand ready to lend trunk support.

How to ask for assistance

If you feel uncomfortable crossing an obstacle or threshold and there is no alternative route, ask for help.

- Ask your helper to push only when your hands are pushing forward on the handrims. If a helper pushes your chair when you are between pushes, you can lose your forward balance.
- As you push forward, your assistant can also push down or pull back slightly on the push handles to unweight the front caster wheels so they will lift up and over obstacles more easily.
- Inform your helper that the bottoms of your foot plates could hit the obstacle. If there is insufficient foot support clearance, have your assistant tip your wheelchair back into a wheelie to cross the obstacle.
- To get into a wheelie position, have your assistant stand behind your wheelchair while holding onto the push handles or back support posts with the pull straps. Have the assistant push down on the handles, back support posts with the pull straps, and/or anti-tip device levers to tip you into a wheelie so your caster wheels can clear the threshold or obstacle. The assistant can rest your wheelchair on his or her knee for additional support.

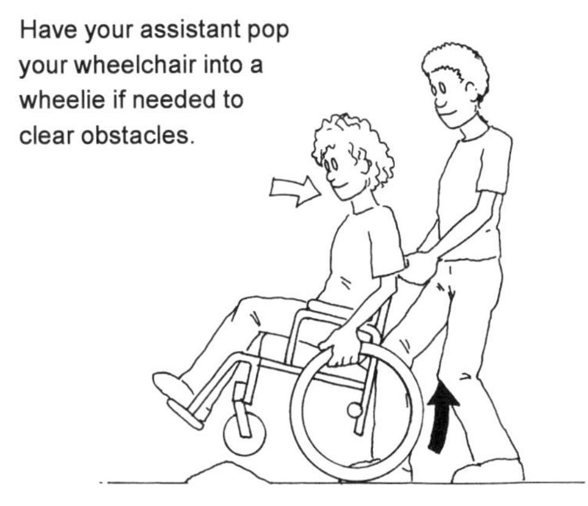
Have your assistant pop your wheelchair into a wheelie if needed to clear obstacles.

- Have the assistant move you forward as you push on the handrims.
- When your caster wheels have cleared the obstacle or threshold, ask the assistant to lower your wheelchair slowly until the caster wheels are back on the floor.
- Lean forward slightly as you push the rear wheels over the obstacle. Ask your helper to hold your shoulders or trunk if you have trouble keeping your balance.
- If you cannot help with the maneuver or have poor balance, use your hands to maintain your trunk balance and have your helper roll your wheelchair over the obstacle. You can hook your arm or arms over the push handles if you need more support.

Section 2.3

Doorways and Tight Environments

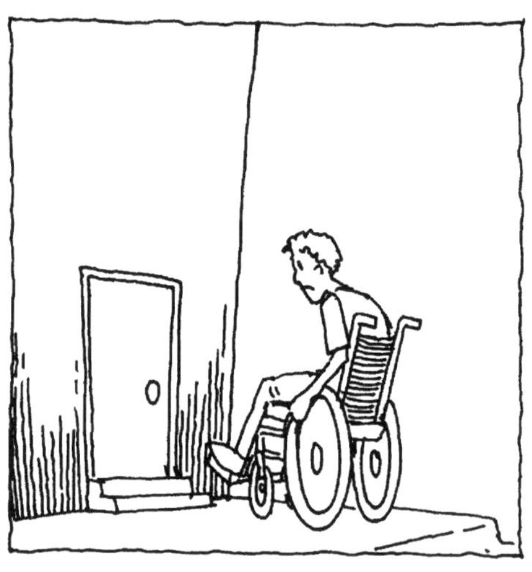

Doorways can pose significant challenges to wheelchair users because they often combine maneuvering within a constricted space, strength to open a door and its latch, and traveling over a threshold. The Americans with Disabilities Act Accessibility Guidelines (ADAAG) have design standards that allow most wheelchair users to negotiate doorways. The ADAAG specifies that doors and gates must have a passageway at least 32 inches wide and should be able to be opened without having to twist or grasp the handle. The ADAAG also states that the threshold should be no more than a quarter-inch in height or a half-inch in height with a beveled transition. (See Appendix A on the Americans With Disabilities Act of 1990 for more information.)

Doors require a certain amount of force to open. Opening a "strong" or "heavy" door set with a lot of tension can be difficult while in a wheelchair because the wheels tend to roll instead of giving you something to brace against. The tension of most doors is adjustable. Exterior doors are set with higher tension than interior ones to keep them from blowing open in the wind. Some interior doors require a lot of force to open because they are fire doors and must not give way against fire drafts. If you encounter a door that is difficult to open, speak to the building's management to see if the tension can be reduced.

If a doorknob or handle is difficult to operate, ask someone to open it for you. Levers are easier to use than round knobs. Some levers are essentially handle extensions that can be installed over existing knobs, while others contain the latch mechanism as well. Door levers are available at hardware stores.

Before learning the skills in this section, you should be able to propel a wheelchair, reach for objects, and cross thresholds. Always have a spotter nearby when trying new skills such as opening doors and moving through tight environments.

How a spotter can help with manually opened doors

When reaching forward for the door handle or crossing the threshold, the rider may fall forward onto his or her lap. Catch the rider at the shoulders to prevent this from happening.

Manual Swinging Doors

With a spotter close by, practice opening and closing doors, and propelling through doorways in bathroom stalls, entryways, and public buildings. If you think you will have difficulty leaning to reach a door handle, ask your spotter to stand to one side and catch you at the trunk if you lose your balance. (See Section 1.7 for more information about bending and reaching.)

Propelling through a doorway usually involves crossing a raised threshold. (See Section 2.2 for more information about crossing thresholds and other obstacles.)

Free-swinging doors

- If the door swings and does not latch shut, approach the door facing forward.
- Make sure the bottom of the door is not glass, which can shatter. Use your foot supports to push the door open. Many doors have kick plates that can be used for this purpose. Contact the door gently so the impact does not hurt your foot or cause your foot supports to go out of adjustment as you push the door open.
- Pay attention to the position of your feet, or you could be nursing a stubbed or broken toe! Approaching the door at an angle from the hinged side of the door will both protect your toes and make it easier to push the door open.

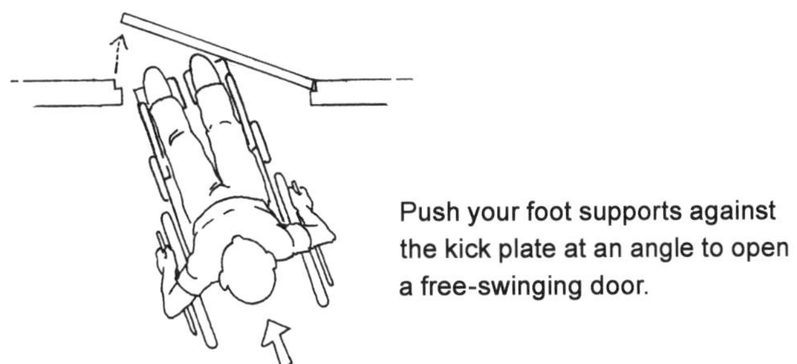

Push your foot supports against the kick plate at an angle to open a free-swinging door.

Doors that open away from you

Going through forward

- As you reach the door, turn slightly to the side. Then facing your wheelchair toward the door handle, reach to the side, unlatch the door, and open it.
- As the door swings open, reposition your wheelchair so both caster wheels touch the threshold or go through the doorway. The ride may be smoother if both caster wheels cross the threshold at the same time. (See Section 2.2 for more information about crossing thresholds and other obstacles.)

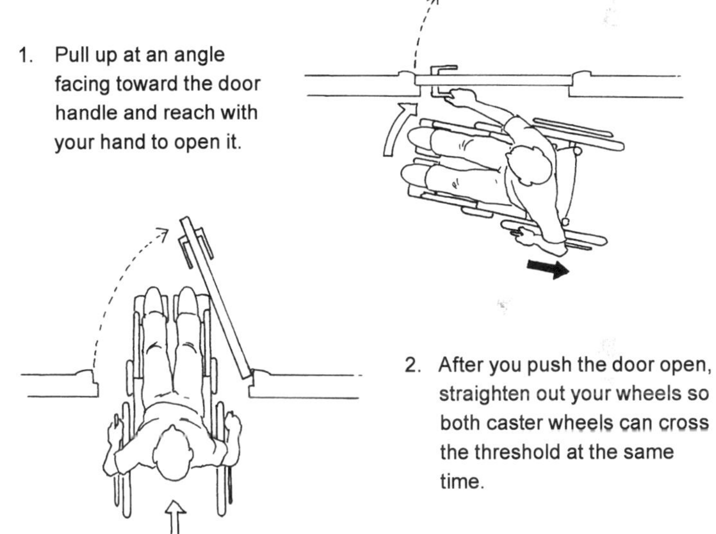

1. Pull up at an angle facing toward the door handle and reach with your hand to open it.
2. After you push the door open, straighten out your wheels so both caster wheels can cross the threshold at the same time.

- If the door is spring loaded, you may need to push the door open with your hand as well as with your foot supports.
- If you have to close the door after you go through it, you should turn around to reach it rather than reaching backwards in order to avoid the risk of tipping over to the rear.
- If the door is not spring loaded, close it with a push.

Going through backward

- Pull up to the door sideways, unlatch it, and push it open.
- Turn so that your back is to the door.
- Quickly pull on your handrims to back through the door. If the door is spring-loaded, it may begin to close but will be stopped by your wheelchair.
- Keep moving backward until your caster wheels have cleared the threshold and you can turn around again.

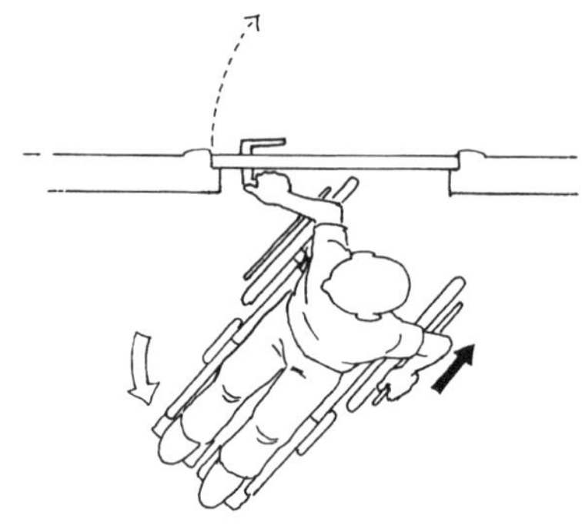

1. Reach to the side to unlatch and push the door open.

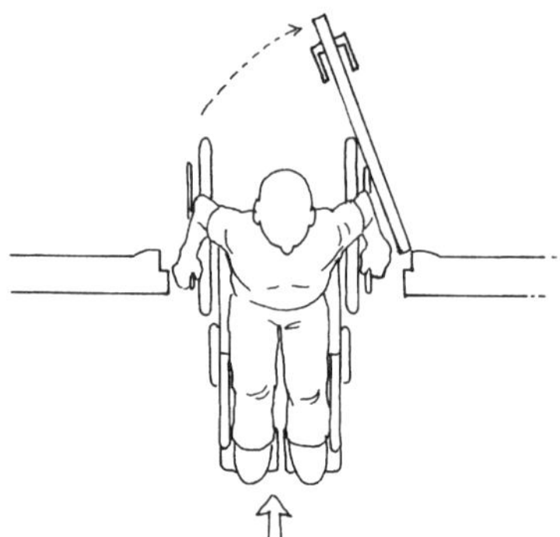

2. Pull backward through the doorway. You can use your rear wheels to push the door open as you go.

Doors that open toward you – with clearance space next to the handle side of the door

- Pull up next to the handle side of the door and reach for the handle.
- Reach sideways to unlatch and open the door with your closest hand.
- Pull the door open, backing up if necessary. You may need to pull once on the handle to open it halfway, and then put your hand on the edge of the door to push it open the rest of the way.
- As the door swings open, pivot into the doorway to block it open. Don't forget about the threshold.
- If the door is spring loaded, it may begin to close, but if you are already on your way through, it should be deflected by your rear wheels and should not be a problem. Continue to move forward through the doorway.

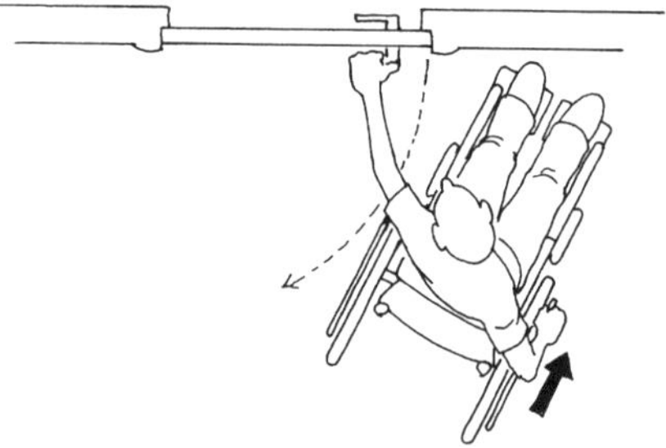

1. You may have to move your wheelchair around the door as you pull it open.

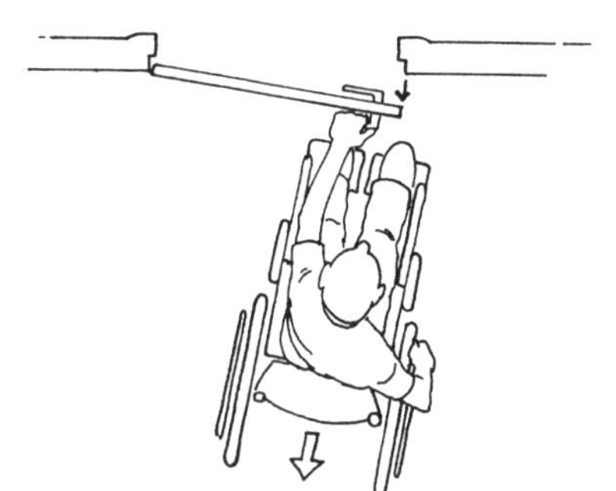

2. Pull the door open to your side or back up as you pull the door open.

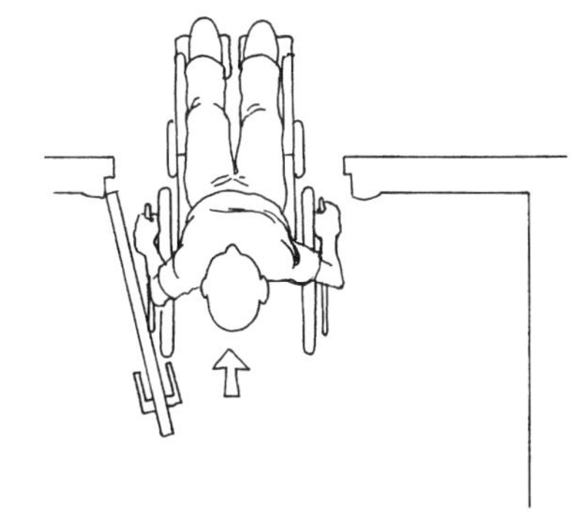

3. Pivot your wheelchair into the doorway opening. Your wheels will prevent a spring-loaded door from closing as you go through.

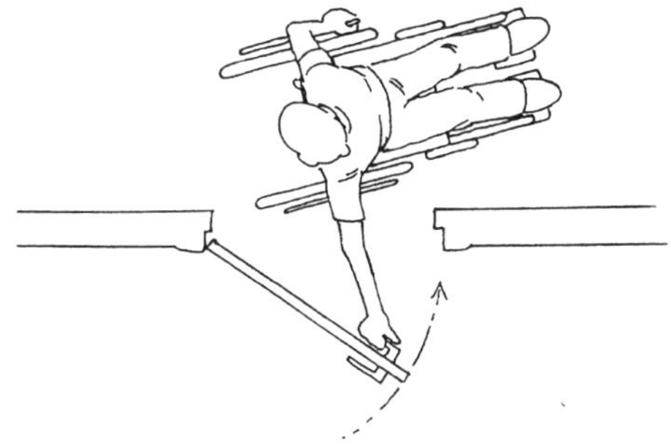

4. Close doors that aren't spring loaded by reaching to the side to grasp the door handle.

Doors that open toward you – that do not have clearance space next to the handle side of the door

Going through forward

- Reach forward and unlatch the door.
- Back up as you pull the door open.
- While it is swinging open, propel your wheelchair forward into the doorway. Don't forget about the threshold.
- A spring loaded door may hit your wheelchair or your rear wheels as you go through.

Going through backward

- Turn your wheelchair so your back is to the door.
- Reach behind you and pull the door open.
- When the door is open wide enough, hold onto the edge of the door to push it open wider.
- Quickly pull on your handrims and/or tires to back through the doorway. The door may begin to close but it will be stopped by your wheelchair. If it prevents you from continuing through the doorway, push it open again.
- Keep moving backward until you have cleared the threshold and can turn forward again.

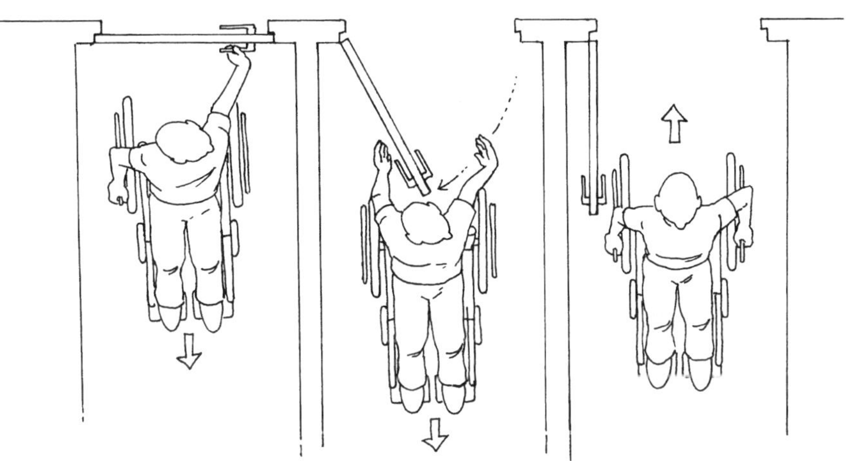

1. Back up to the door and grasp the handle with the nearest hand.
2. Move forward to open the door.
3. Back up slightly to hold the door open with one wheel and then back through the opening.

Manual Sliding Doors

Manual sliding doors slide instead of swing open. Exterior sliding glass and screen doors usually ride on floor tracks. Floor tracks can be more difficult to cross than conventional thresholds because they are taller and have sharper edges. Transition ramps can be purchased for sliding doors that you use all of the time in your home. (See Section 2.2 for more information about crossing thresholds and other obstacles.) Drop-offs on sliding door thresholds can be hazardous and can cause you to tip forward out of your chair.

"Pocket" sliding doors, usually found inside, ride on an overhead track and do not have a raised threshold to obstruct your passage. Indoor "pocket" doors should not present a problem once they are open because there is usually no raised threshold.

While practicing, have a spotter prevent you from losing your balance when sliding heavier doors.

- To open the door, it is usually easiest to rotate your wheelchair until you are almost parallel with the door.
- Some people find it easier to pull the door open. Others find it easier to turn around and push the door open.
- Open the door until it is wide enough to pass through. You can grab the door frame with your other hand to help stabilize yourself while opening the door.

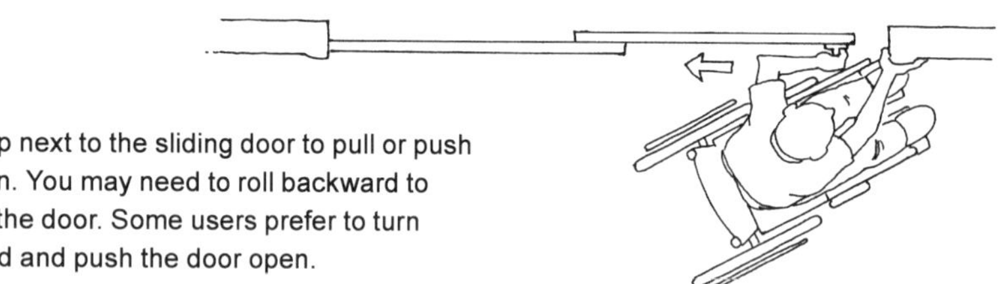

Pull up next to the sliding door to pull or push it open. You may need to roll backward to open the door. Some users prefer to turn around and push the door open.

- Reposition your wheelchair so both caster wheels cross the threshold at the same time. (See Section 2.2 for more information about crossing thresholds and obstacles.) Some people like to hold onto the door and door frame as their rear wheels pass over the threshold.
- After you pass through the doorway, rotate into a good position to slide the door shut by pushing or pulling on the door. If there is a larger drop off on the other side of the door threshold, some users prefer to roll backwards through the doorway while holding onto the door frame for stability. Have a spotter behind you the first time you try this.

Helpful Hint

If you have trouble using a particular door, look for an alternate entrance. You may need to ask someone familiar with the building. To avoid such situations, phone the establishment before your visit to inquire about access.

Doors in a Sequence

Many buildings, particularly in colder climates, have entrances with two doors in quick succession. Typically, there will be one swinging door, a short space, and then a second swinging door. If there is enough space for you to pass through the first door and reposition yourself for the second, you can follow the recommendations for passing through conventional swinging doors.

Problems arise when the doors are spaced so closely that you cannot pass all the way through the first door and into the space before you need to open the second. Problems also occur when one or both doors open toward you and block the clear space that you need for your wheelchair to maneuver. As the doors swing, they create obstacles you must work to avoid.

Before attempting doors in a sequence, you should know how to open a single manual-swinging door. Always have a spotter nearby as you practice in case you need help or get trapped between the doors. Hotels, post offices and other public buildings are good places to practice opening doors in a sequence.

- Open the first door using the skills listed under "Manual Swinging Doors."
- If the second door opens into the space between the doors and the space is short, try to use your wheelchair to prop the first door open. This will give you room to back up through the first doorway and position your wheelchair to open and pass through the second doorway.

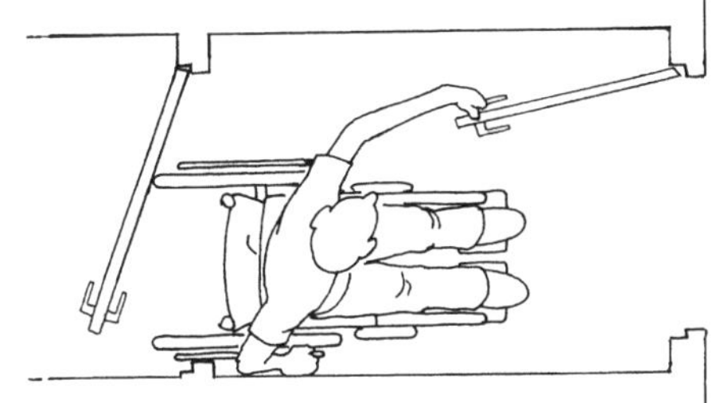

Use the rear wheels to prop open the first door as you open the second.

How to ask for assistance

- If opening doors is difficult, ask someone to help you by opening and holding one or both doors for you to propel through. (You may need to plan how to hold the first door open while your assistant changes position to open the second door.)
- If you need help crossing the threshold, see Section 2.2.

Double-Leaf Doors

A double-leaf door is made up of two narrow swinging doors that open in the center. Saloon style and French doors are considered double-leaf doors.

Double-leaf doors are fairly rare. However, if you spend a lot of time in a place with them, take a few minutes to practice with a spotter.

If the door handle is outside, beyond your reach, ask a spotter to stand to one side of your wheelchair. The spotter should be ready to catch you if you lose your balance while leaning forward to open the latch. If opening the door or doors is difficult, ask someone to hold one or both open as you propel through.

Open double-leaf doors using the skills for manual swinging doors. If you need help crossing the threshold, see Section 2.2.

Narrow Doors

To pass unassisted through a door that is too narrow for your chair, you may have to do a series of transfers. Although it is usually easier to find a different route, you may have no choice but to do this. These situations sometimes arise in hotel rooms where the door to the bathroom is narrow and the bathroom space is small. First, try to get help from maintenance to remove the door from its hinges. It is fairly easy to do and many hotels will install a curtain or put up a sheet for privacy if the door is removed. If the doorway is still too narrow for you to enter, transfer into a chair placed inside the bathroom and then bring your folded or disassembled wheelchair inside if necessary.

Practice on doors of different widths that swing in different directions. When practicing, have a spotter assist you if you get stuck or need help.

Entering with the use of a four-legged chair

- Put a four-legged chair on the other side of the doorway.
- Position your wheelchair for a transfer and apply the wheel locks.
- If possible, remove your foot support nearest the four-legged chair or swing your foot support out of the way before positioning the chair.
- Place one hand on the chair while keeping the other on the arm support or seat rail of your wheelchair to steady yourself.
- Transfer to the four-legged chair.

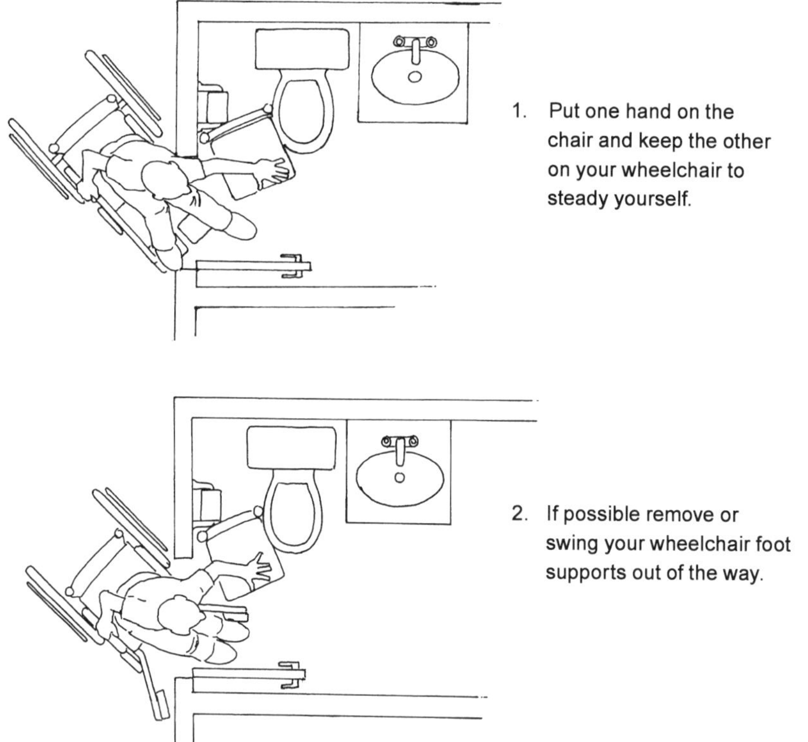

1. Put one hand on the chair and keep the other on your wheelchair to steady yourself.
2. If possible remove or swing your wheelchair foot supports out of the way.

- If you need your wheelchair inside the bathroom, fold or disassemble your wheelchair to pull it through the door.
- Transfer back into your wheelchair.

Entering without using a four-legged chair

- Position your wheelchair to facilitate a safe transfer to the floor. (Some people prefer to position their wheelchair as close to the doorway as possible, while others prefer to transfer clear of the doorway.)
- Transfer from your wheelchair to the floor and pull yourself through the doorway. You may need to sit on your wheelchair cushion as you slide or scoot across the floor to protect your skin.
- If you need your wheelchair inside the bathroom, pull your wheelchair through the doorway. You may have to remove the wheels or fold the chair to fit it through the doorway.
- Transfer back into your wheelchair once it is reassembled. You may choose not to bring your wheelchair into the space if you will not need it.

Entering by removing one rear wheel

One way to reduce the width of your wheelchair is to remove one wheel. This is most easily done on chairs with "quick release" wheels. Push the button in the center of the quick release wheel while pulling the wheel away from the frame to remove it. Not all wheelchairs have quick release wheels.

- Have your assistant support the back of your wheelchair by holding the push handles or back support posts with the pull straps.
- Shift your weight forward and to the opposite side of the chair from the wheel you will be removing.

- Remove the wheel on the opposite side. If you feel uncomfortable removing the wheel yourself, have your assistant remove the wheel for you. Have your assistant hold your wheelchair level as they roll you through the doorway on three wheels.
- When you are through the narrow space, replace the wheel.
- Wait until the wheel is replaced before sitting upright.

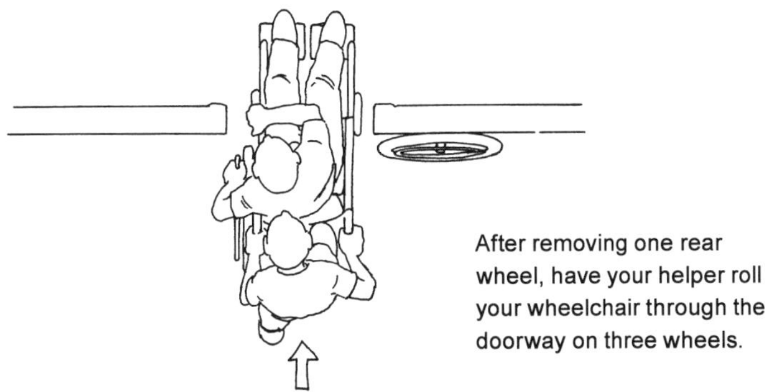

After removing one rear wheel, have your helper roll your wheelchair through the doorway on three wheels.

Entering by removing both rear wheels

- Have a strong assistant support the back of your wheelchair by holding the push handles or back support posts with the pull straps, lifting the rear wheels off the ground. If you have anti-tip wheels, install them so your wheelchair can roll on these wheels after removing the main wheels.
- Shift your weight forward.
- Have another assistant remove both rear wheels.
- Have your strong assistant roll you though the doorway on your front casters. If you have anti-tip devices with wheels, your assistant will be able to roll you through the doorway on them.
- This technique can also be used to get down the aisle of an aircraft as shown in Section 4.7 Transportation, if you have a strong assistant.
- When you have reached the other side, have your strong assistant replace the wheels before sitting upright.

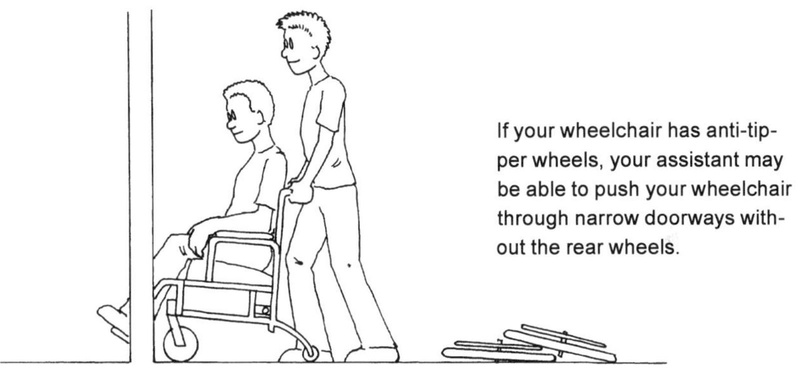

If your wheelchair has anti-tipper wheels, your assistant may be able to push your wheelchair through narrow doorways without the rear wheels.

Automatic Doors

Automatic doors are usually found at supermarkets and medical facilities. Since the passing of the American's with Disabilities Act, automatic doors are becoming more common. These doors are very convenient, since they do the work of opening the door for you. Some are operated by stepping, or wheeling, onto a sensor pad that is slightly higher than the ground. The soft or ribbed surface on many sensor pads can be tricky to cross.

Many automatic doors are triggered by an optical sensor aimed at an area in front of the door. If a person enters the area scanned by the sensor, the door opens. If the door does not open, look around the door frame for a sensor. Approach the door again, this time crossing the sensor's path. You may need to wave your hand or arm above your head to trigger an optical sensor that is aimed too high for a wheelchair rider.

You may be moving faster than a person who is walking when you approach an automatic door. Slow to "walking speed" to give the door time to swing or slide open.

While these doors are designed to stay open as you pass through, some sensors and timing devices may still cause the doors to close on you.

Revolving Doors and Turnstiles

Revolving doors and turnstiles are often difficult and sometimes impossible to negotiate in a wheelchair. An alternative entrance should be offered in places with revolving doors and turnstiles. In many places, a door attendant can unlock the revolving doors to create a conventional entrance. If an alternative entrance is not available, you may have to negotiate the turnstile or revolving doors to enter the building.

Turnstiles that can be opened like gates should not pose a problem for you, but if the turnstile cannot be operated like a gate, and the arms of the turnstile lock in each position, you may get trapped while trying to pass through. Watch a few people pass through it to determine if your wheelchair will make it.

Watch a few revolutions of revolving doors to get a sense of the timing required to use them, since some are faster than others and some have bigger openings than others. If the doors do not spin automatically, ask an assistant to spin the doors so you can concentrate on rolling your wheelchair. Be aware that some revolving doors can sense how close you are to the door and moving too close to the door panel in front, or behind you, will stop the doors.

Revolving doors that rotate in a large oval may be able to accommodate wheelchairs more easily but still require care and caution to negotiate safely.

Doors with Objects Around Them

Although the Americans with Disabilities Act Accessibility Guidelines require doors to have a certain amount of open space around them, obstacles such as trash cans, free-standing signs, and potted plants are frequently placed alongside doors. These can make reaching the doorknob and opening and closing the door difficult. Ways to cope with such objects include:

- Pushing the obstacles out of the way with your foot supports.
- Asking someone to move the obstacles for you.
- Informing the business establishment's management. They may not have recognized the problem and may be willing to correct it.

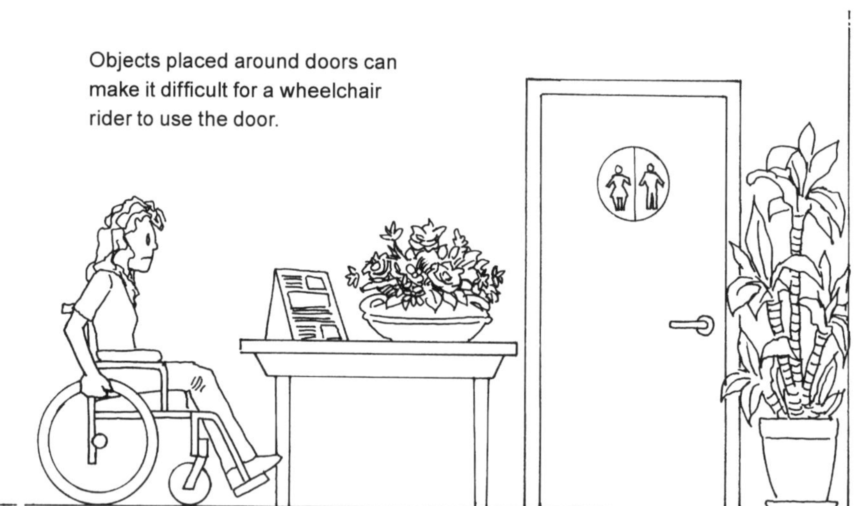

Objects placed around doors can make it difficult for a wheelchair rider to use the door.

Tight Environments

A lack of floor space, objects on walls, and furniture, such as tables, can all limit your maneuvering space. Narrow hallways, van interiors, small apartments, and household bathrooms can leave wheelchair users with very little room to maneuver. Because it can be so difficult to use a wheelchair in tight environments, it is often a good idea to find alternative routes or spaces to use.

- Remember, if you have small front caster wheels and a lower front end, you may be able to move the front portion of your wheelchair closer to certain objects, such as bathroom sinks and/or tables. Look underneath any object you plan to roll under to be sure your knees and/or legs will not hit any sharp edges. Many round tables in restaurants have portions of their tables that fold, transforming them into square tables. The folding mechanisms on these tables are metal and hang down underneath and can be very sharp.
- Since your rear wheels project behind the back support of your wheelchair, it can be difficult to backup to many objects.
- Remember that your caster wheels must be in the correct trail position for the front of the chair to change directions. (See Section 1.5 for more information about caster wheel management.) This often makes maneuvering in small spaces difficult because it takes a little bit of space for the casters to pivot to the required trailing direction.
- Backing into a small space often puts you in a better position to maneuver once you are inside the space.
- Removing the foot supports reduces your wheelchair's overall length and might make it easier to turn around. Try not to bump your feet or get them caught in your caster wheels. Removing one foot support and crossing that foot over the opposite ankle may also help you complete a maneuver within a tight space.

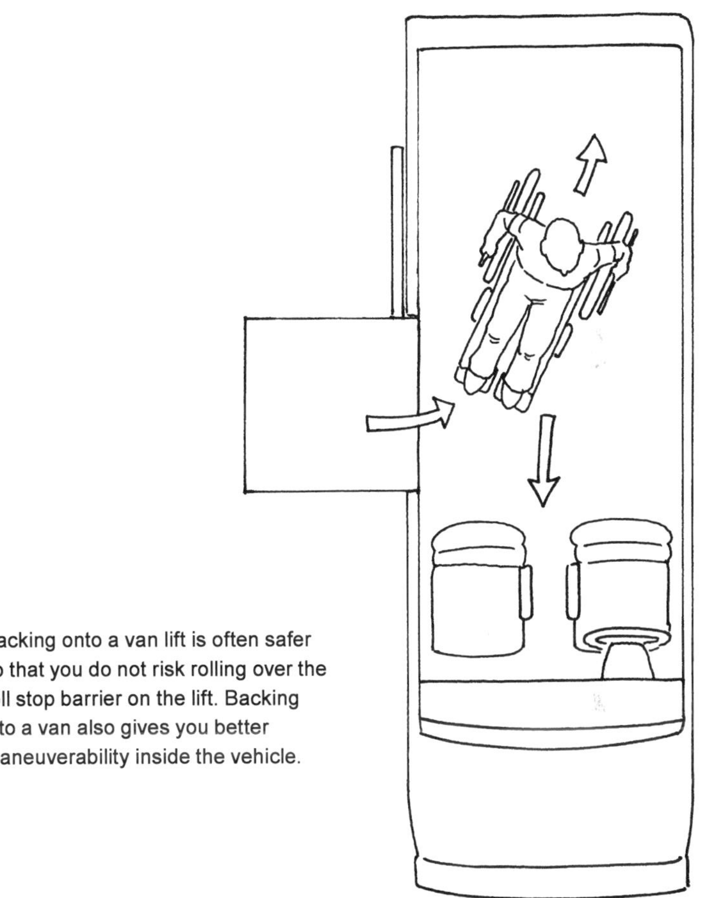

Backing onto a van lift is often safer so that you do not risk rolling over the roll stop barrier on the lift. Backing into a van also gives you better maneuverability inside the vehicle.

Turning in Narrow Hallways

Sometimes hallways or other spaces are so narrow that you cannot turn your wheelchair around. You may need to back up to a wider portion of the hallway or perform a multi-point turn.

Backing up

- Propel your wheelchair forward or backward until you reach a space wide enough for you to turn around.
- Be sure to look behind you for other people or obstacles.

Three-point turn

- Make sure the hallway is a little wider than your wheelchair's length.
- Check for oncoming traffic and obstacles behind you.
- If the path is clear, pull to one side of the hallway.
- Turn the chair sharply and roll toward the opposite wall in a tight diagonal.
- When you can't go any farther in that direction, back up at a diagonal and continue the turn.
- When you cannot go any farther in that direction, go forward.
- Continue moving back and forth to complete the turn.

Hopping turn

Some people can perform a hop turn by gripping their tires and hopping to move the rear of the chair sideways without moving forward or backward. This pivoting maneuver can also be used to hop sideways in close quarters.

Hopping can help you maneuver in very tight quarters.

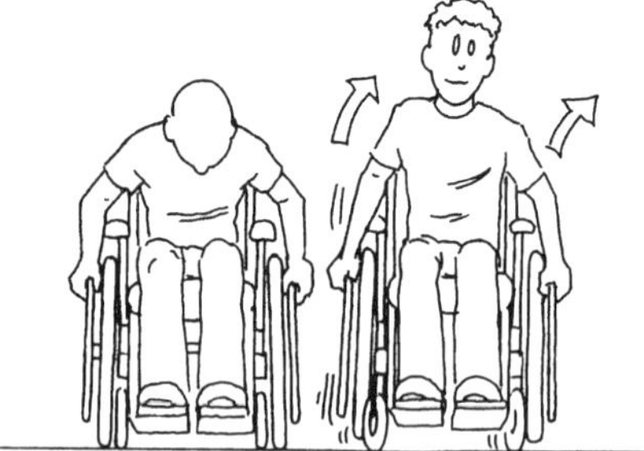

Turning into a doorway from a narrow hallway

Pull to the far side of the hallway, opposite the door, before turning. The extra space will permit you to complete more of the turn and reduce the likelihood of needing to make a 3-point turn.

Sometimes removing the foot support on the opposite side of the chair from the direction you are turning can help when moving from very narrow hallways into tight doorways. Cross the leg without a foot support over the opposite leg's ankle and then make the turn. For example, if you are turning left, remove the right foot support.

Removing a foot support and crossing that leg over your other foot can reduce your width enough to turn out of a narrow hallway.

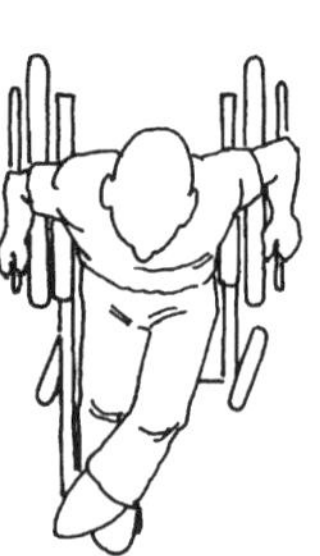

Section 2.4

Rough Terrain

If you're active, you will encounter many surfaces that are difficult to cross in your wheelchair. Rough terrain such as uneven asphalt, grass, mud, sand, cobblestones, outdoor recreation trails, and wooden planking are common surfaces that require special skills to cross. Practice crossing different surfaces to get a feel for which ones you can negotiate independently.

If bumps on rough terrain jolt you out of position, reposition yourself once you are back on smooth ground or when you can no longer propel yourself safely and/or efficiently. Traveling slowly will make the ride less rough.

Larger, softer, and wider tires make travel over rough surfaces and obstacles easier, but can be sluggish on smooth surfaces such as concrete or linoleum. (Section 1.2 discusses how tires affect performance.)

When learning to travel across rough terrain, have a spotter ready to catch you and prevent you from falling. Examine the surface ahead to anticipate upcoming obstacles such as grooves between tiles that might catch your caster wheels, throw rugs that can bunch up beneath your wheels, and changes in surface type that may throw you off balance.

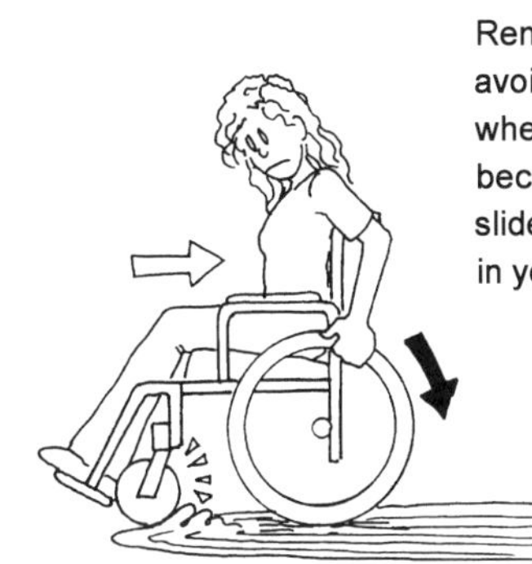

Remove or avoid loose rugs whenever possible because they can slide and get caught in your wheels.

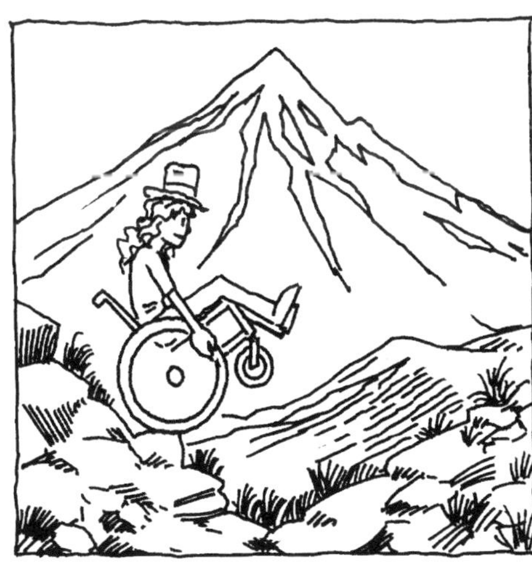

Before attempting to learn rough terrain skills, you should be able to propel a wheelchair forward and backward, and cross thresholds. The ability to move forward in a wheelie will give you maximum mobility over rough surfaces.

Start practicing on carpet and tile, working up to hard, uneven surfaces such as buckling sidewalks, and finally attempting softer surfaces such as grass, gravel-covered dirt, and natural surface outdoor recreation trails. Start slowly, and gradually increase your speed on each surface; there may be an optimum speed that is fast enough for momentum to help carry you but slow enough to maintain your balance. If a spotter is helping you negotiate rough terrain, use a spotter strap as described and explained in Section 1.9 Wheelies.

Hard, Uneven Surfaces

It is generally easiest to move across hard, uneven surfaces in a wheelie. However, start practicing to cross rough terrain on all four wheels with a spotter before graduating to a wheelie position. Remember that the faster you travel, the harder the fall you could experience if you lose your balance.

Move across the wooden planks of decks, piers, and boardwalks perpendicular to the boards so your caster wheels do not get stuck in the space between the boards. When surfaces change, such as linoleum giving way to carpet, a small step may be created. (See Section 2.2 for more information about crossing these obstacles.) To avoid catching your caster wheels in tile grout, cross perpendicular or diagonal to the grooves.

Riding over bumps can trigger muscle spasms, which could make it difficult to stay upright and balanced. If you have spasticity, always try to avoid rough terrain or ride slowly over bumps.

Soft Surfaces

Whenever possible, cross soft surfaces in a wheelie. This will reduce the amount of wheel drag you experience. Maintain forward momentum when crossing soft surfaces to keep your wheels from sinking. If you do not cross in a wheelie, keeping your caster wheels aligned with the rear wheels may help keep you from getting stuck. (See Section 1.5 for more information about caster wheel management.)

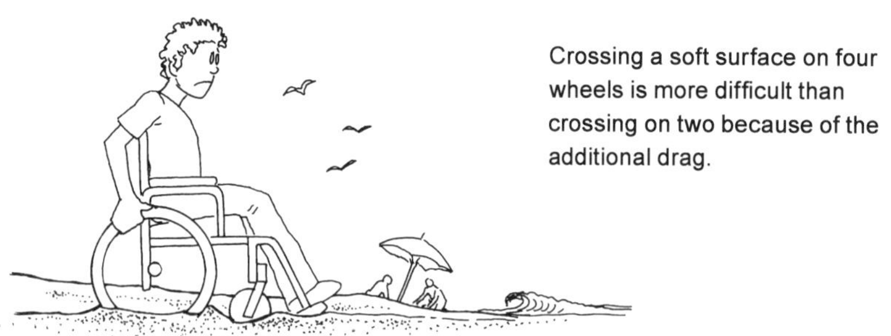

Crossing a soft surface on four wheels is more difficult than crossing on two because of the additional drag.

Crossing on Four Wheels

Crossing soft or rough terrain on four wheels is a matter of simple forward (or not so simple) propulsion. If you are moving too quickly over rough terrain, the caster wheels may catch on the surface, causing your wheelchair to stop suddenly, throwing your body forward and possibly out of the chair.

How to ask for assistance

If you think you will need help crossing an uneven surface, ask someone to give you a hand.

- Have your assistant stand behind your wheelchair with his/her hands on the push handles.
- Ask your assistant to push forward on the push handles while you are propelling on the handrims.
- As you push forward, your assistant can also push down or pull back slightly on the push handles to unweight the front caster wheels so they will lift up and over obstacles more easily.
- Sometimes it is easier and safer to have someone pull you backwards across the surface, especially if the slope is downhill.
- If you have a climbing sling or a piece of rope or webbing, you can attach it near the top of the front caster on the frame of your wheelchair and have your assistant move to the front of the chair to pull up and forward. This will keep weight off of your casters and help pull you forward at the

same time. (see Section 4.4 Hiking.) With a climbing sling or strap on each side of your wheelchair, you can have two assistants help you through really soft surfaces such as sand or snow. You can also ask one assistant to be in front of the chair and one to be behind your chair.

How a spotter can help

- Walk next to the wheelchair user.
- Be ready to catch the rider at the shoulder if he or she loses balance.

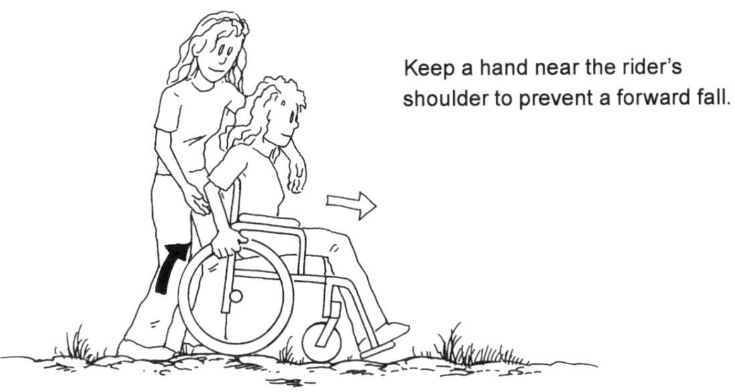

Keep a hand near the rider's shoulder to prevent a forward fall.

- Stand behind the wheelchair if you need to help push. Pushing down on the push handles will unweight the casters.

Crossing in a Wheelie

Whenever possible, cross rough terrain in a wheelie to reduce drag and keep your caster wheels out of ruts.

- Pop a wheelie and roll forward in a wheelie position. Progress slowly over the surface at first. Once you are comfortable and confident, you can try going faster until you find a speed that works best for you.
- If it becomes difficult to maintain the wheelie for the duration of the rough surface, you may need to drop out of the wheelie to rest before proceeding.
- If your wheels get stuck along the way, rock the chair forward and back to gain enough traction to continue.

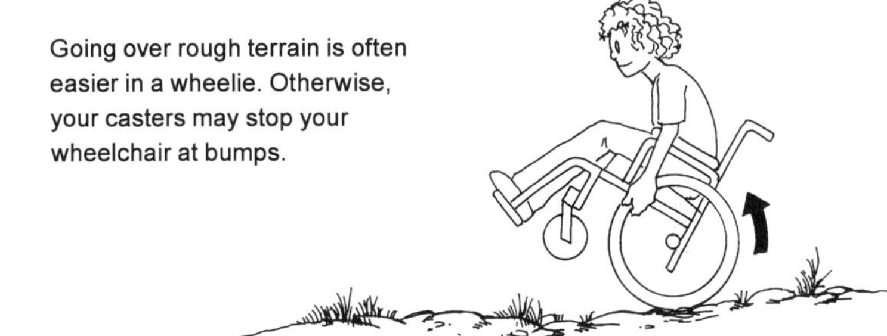

Going over rough terrain is often easier in a wheelie. Otherwise, your casters may stop your wheelchair at bumps.

How to ask for assistance

- Together with your assistant, tip your wheelchair into a wheelie. (See Section 1.9 for more information about wheelies.)
- Ask your assistant to assist with keeping your wheelchair in the wheelie position by holding onto your wheelchair's push handles or back support posts with the pull straps.
- Sometimes it is easier to have someone pull you backwards across a surface in a wheelie.
- When you have cleared the uneven or soft terrain, ask your assistant to lower the caster wheels to the ground.
- Rather than crossing in a wheelie, if you have a climbing sling or a piece of rope or webbing, you can attach it near the top of the front caster on the frame of your wheelchair and have your assistant move to the front of the chair to pull up and forward.

How a spotter can help

- Walk next to the wheelchair user.
- Be ready to prevent the wheelchair user from falling forward out of the wheelchair if it stops suddenly.
- Be ready to prevent the wheelchair user from tipping over backwards in his or her wheelchair. With the permission of the wheelchair user you can help keep the wheelchair balanced in a wheelie by holding onto the push handles or the back of the wheelchair with a loose grip.

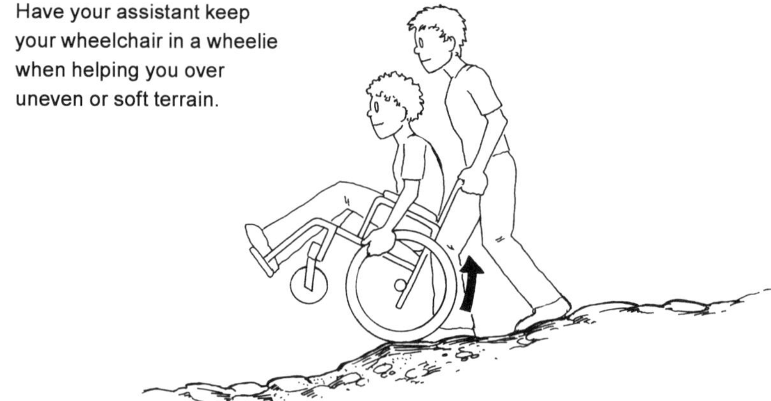

Have your assistant keep your wheelchair in a wheelie when helping you over uneven or soft terrain.

Section 2.5

Ramps

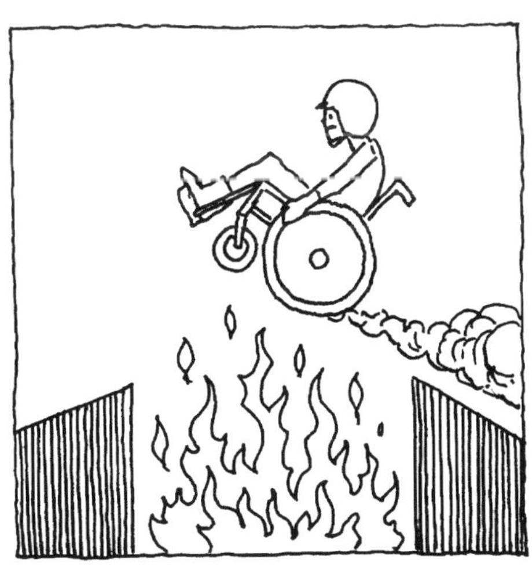

According to the Americans with Disabilities Act Accessibility Guidelines (ADAAG), a standard ramp should have a grade no steeper than 1:12. This means that for every one inch of rise (change in height), there should be 12 inches of run (change in length). This is sometimes referred to as an 8% grade or slope. Using this formula, a ramp going to a platform with two 8-inch steps (creates a total of 16 inches of rise) should be 16 feet long. A standard ramp is gradual enough for many people to climb safely, but each individual's limits are different. Some people may not be able to manage a ramp this steep, while others can handle much steeper ramps. With experimentation, you will learn how steep a ramp you can negotiate alone. Always use a spotter when practicing on ramps and when climbing a steep ramp for the first time. You can practice on public ramps and you may also find using a ramp with a railing easier. Climb increasingly steeper ramps until you find one that causes your front caster wheels to lift off the ground. Experience the loss of stability, and visually remember the steepness of the slope that caused this to happen. Obtain assistance before climbing slopes this steep or steeper in the future.

Before learning the skills in this section, you should be able to propel a wheelchair forward and backward, and maintain a seated position when your balance is challenged. You will be able to perform more techniques and negotiate steeper slopes if you can pop a wheelie and move forward and backward in the wheelie position.

Going Up a Ramp

Put your anti-tip devices down in a functional position before ascending a ramp, because if the ramp is steep, your wheelchair may tip over backward. Sometimes anti-tip devices catch at the beginning of a ramp. If you must disengage the anti-tip devices, move slowly, lean forward, use an assistant, and be extra careful.

A backpack or other gear on the back of your wheelchair changes your center of gravity and will cause you to tip backward more easily. When you have a backpack on your wheelchair you will find that your chair may be less balanced going up ramps.

When you roll up a ramp, you have to re-grip the wheels quickly in between pushes or your wheelchair will roll backwards in between pushes. Devices called hill-climbers can be attached to prevent your wheelchair from rolling backwards between pushes as you travel up grades, hills or ramps. These are especially helpful if you are not strong enough to maintain your momentum between pushes going up the ramps you normally encounter.

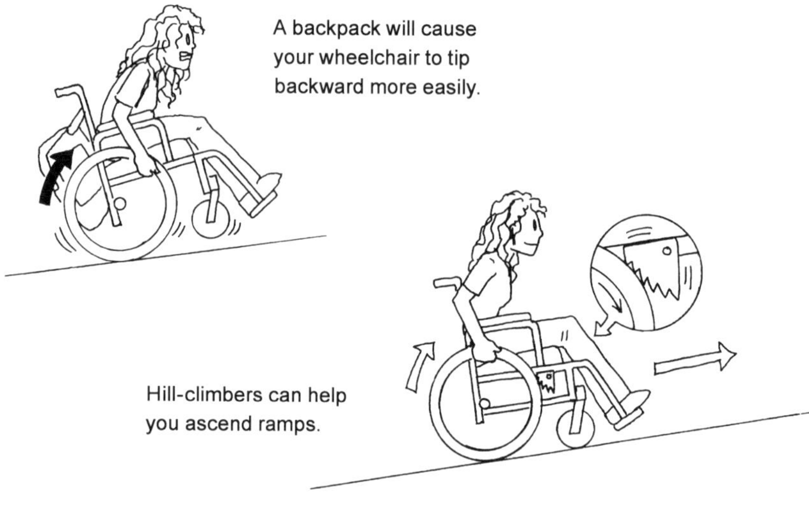
A backpack will cause your wheelchair to tip backward more easily.

Hill-climbers can help you ascend ramps.

Going up forward

Basic technique

- Propel forward onto the ramp.
- Lean forward to counteract the tendency of your wheelchair to tip backward.
- Some people prefer propelling up the ramp with long strokes originating far back on the handrims. Other people can obtain more momentum and power with short, quick propulsion strokes. Experiment with both to see which technique works best for you.
- If you start slowing down, try alternating hands on the handrims. Push first on one side and then on the other. This way one of your hands is always on your wheel preventing it from rolling backwards. This technique may not work on steeper ramps. (See Section 1.8 for more information about this propulsion technique.)
- Turn your wheelchair sideways to the ramp slope and lean into the hill if you need to rest.

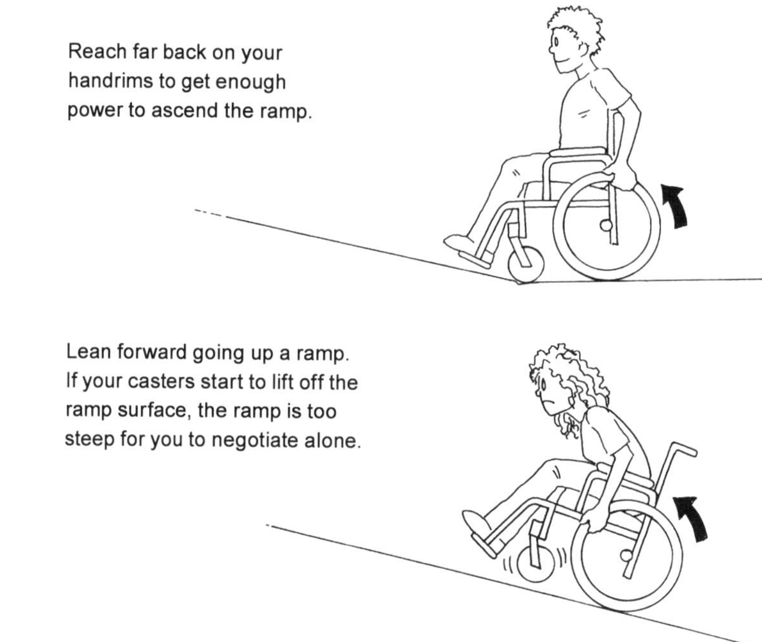
Reach far back on your handrims to get enough power to ascend the ramp.

Lean forward going up a ramp. If your casters start to lift off the ramp surface, the ramp is too steep for you to negotiate alone.

Using momentum

- Gather as much speed as you can before you reach the base of the ramp so your momentum can help propel you up the ramp.
- Propel quickly up the ramp until you start running out of strength.
- Turn the chair sideways to the ramp slope and lean into the hill to rest.

Use momentum to help you ascend the ramp. If you get tired midway, stop and rest with your wheelchair turned perpendicular to the ramp slope.

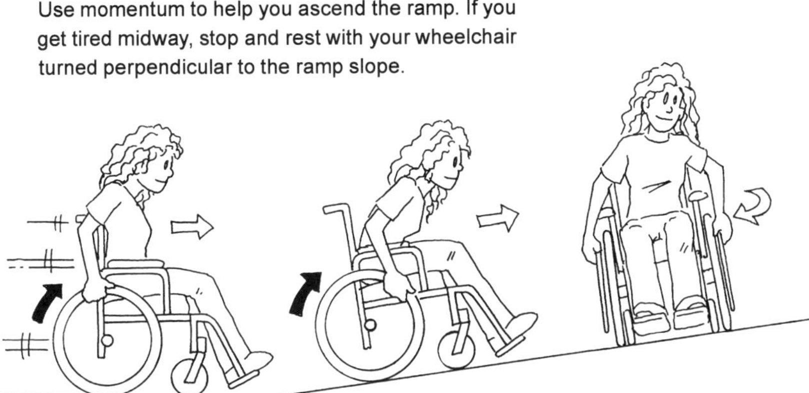

Using handrails

- If there is at least one handrail on the ramp, you can pull yourself up by pushing on one handrim and pulling on a handrail with the other hand.
- If there are two handrails on the ramp and you can reach them both, you can use them to pull yourself up the ramp.

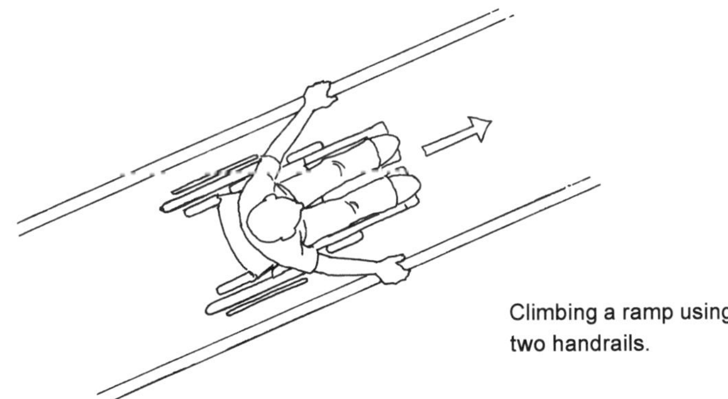

Climbing a ramp using two handrails.

How a spotter can help

- Walk behind the wheelchair user and place your hands close to the push handles or back support posts with the pull straps. Try not to influence the movement of the wheelchair.
- Prevent the wheelchair from tipping over backward.

The spotter should walk behind your wheelchair with hands close to the push handles.

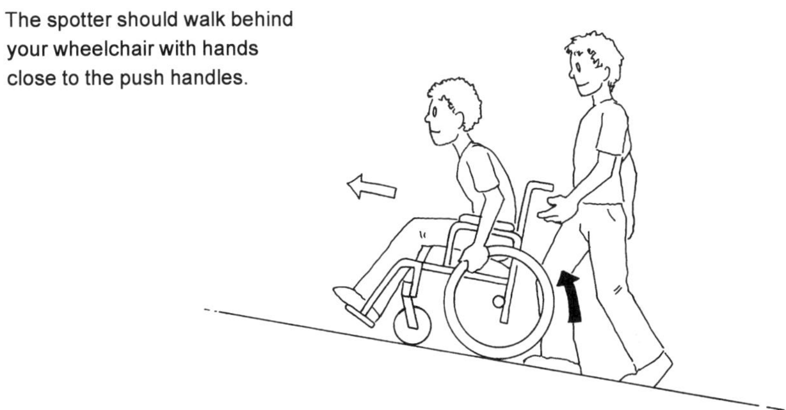

Going up backward

Some people, especially those who propel their wheelchairs with their feet, find it easier to travel up ramps backward. Before going up, make sure the ramp is wide enough for your wheelchair, and check for hazards such as uneven surfaces, obstacles, unprotected drop-offs, and oncoming traffic.

- Just before the base of the ramp, turn your wheelchair around so your rear wheels are next to the base of the ramp.
- Propel your wheelchair backward by pulling back on the handrims.
- Lean backward into the hill.
- If you also propel with your feet, walk them up the hill to push your wheelchair.
- At the top, check behind you for oncoming traffic and obstacles before turning around and proceeding forward.

How a spotter can help

- Stay downhill and to the side of the wheelchair user.
- Prevent the rider from falling forward out of the chair.

How to ask for assistance

When you find a steep ramp you cannot climb independently, ask for assistance. Remember the visual slope of ramps that cause you to lose your stability.

- Ask your assistant to push you using your push handles or the back of your wheelchair. Your assistant should also keep your wheelchair from tipping backward.
- Push forward on your handrims at the same time.

Going Down a Ramp

Before descending a ramp, always check for obstacles such as cracks and level changes. Also examine the base of the ramp for any obstacles that you will need to cross, such as drainage grates.

- Shift your weight back (toward the top of the hill) when going down ramps.
- Proceed slowly to maintain control. As you get more comfortable and confident with ramps, you will be able to increase your speed and remain safe.
- Apply pressure to the handrims to reduce your speed.
- If the foot supports contacted the ramp at the start of the climb, they will contact the ground coming back down at the bottom of the ramp. If you're moving slowly, you will be less likely to get thrown out of your chair if your foot supports contact the bottom of the ramp.

Always practice descending ramps using a spotter. Malls, medical facilities, and other public places generally have good practice ramps. Move forward down ramps of increasing steepness with a spotter until you can no longer descend independently with confidence. Always obtain assistance when you do not feel comfortable descending a ramp independently.

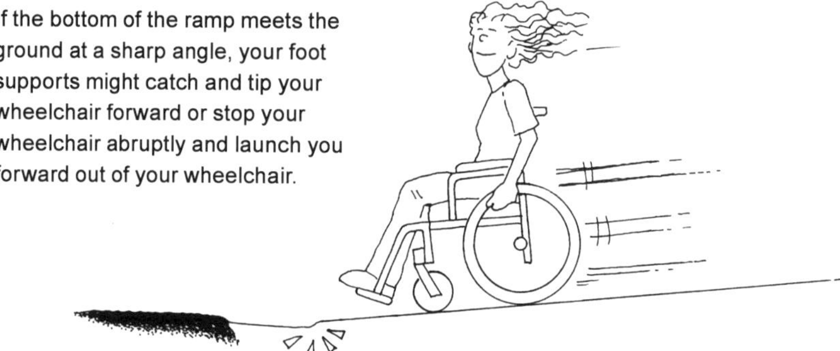

If the bottom of the ramp meets the ground at a sharp angle, your foot supports might catch and tip your wheelchair forward or stop your wheelchair abruptly and launch you forward out of your wheelchair.

Going down a ramp forward

On four wheels

Start practicing ramp descents by going down on four wheels.

- Examine the ramp for obstacles.
- Propel your wheelchair forward onto the ramp, shifting your weight back to avoid falling forward out of the chair.
- Proceed slowly to maintain control.
- Keep your arms forward with your hands cupped on the handrims.
- Apply pressure on the handrims by squeezing your hands to reduce your speed.

How to ask for assistance

- Ask your assistant to hold onto the push handles or back support posts with the pull straps as you move down the ramp.

- Shift your weight back to avoid falling forward out of your chair.
- Your assistant can pull back on the push handles to reduce your speed. Be sure your assistant uses leg rather than back strength. (See Section 5.1 for more information on how to prevent back injuries.)
- If you think you will have trouble maintaining upright sitting balance, have your assistant turn you around and roll you down the ramp backwards. This is always advisable on really steep ramps.

How a spotter can help

- Remain in front and to the side of the wheelchair user.
- Prevent the wheelchair user from toppling forward out of the chair.
- Be sure to stay out of the wheelchair user's path of travel.

Have your spotter walk in front and to the side of your wheelchair when descending a ramp.

You can push forward against your spotter with one hand if your spotter leans back into the hill to provide resistance to your forward movement.

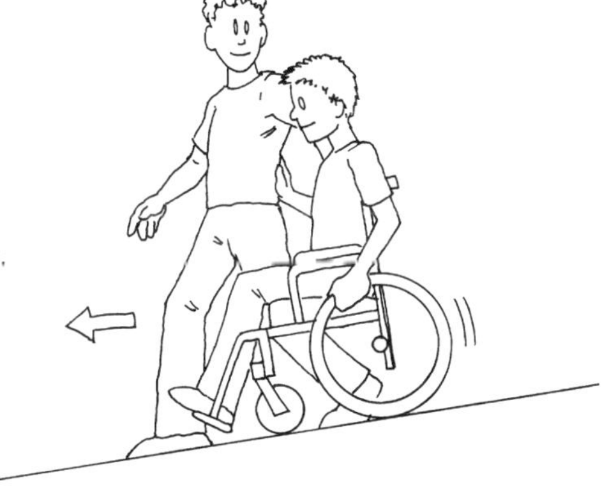

Going down a ramp using a wheelie

Traveling down steeper ramps on four wheels could cause you to fall forward. Traveling down steeper ramps in a wheelie can help you avoid this problem. In a wheelie, your weight is back and you will be less likely to fall forward out of your wheelchair.

- Check the ramp for any obstacles.
- Facing the ramp, pop a wheelie.
- Maintaining wheelie position, roll forward onto the ramp.
- Allow the handrims to slide through your grasp, applying more pressure to reduce speed or reducing pressure to increase speed.
- More gripping pressure will reduce your speed while less gripping pressure will increase your speed.
- Some users prefer to lean back, which means they do not have to pop their wheelie very high. Others prefer to lean or flex forward resulting in a higher wheelie. Some users feel that the higher wheelie gives them more visibility and control going down the ramp.
- Come out of the wheelie after you are back on level ground at a landing or the bottom of the ramp.

Some users prefer to flex forward, resulting in a higher wheelie so they have more visibility going down the ramp.

How to instruct a spotter to help you

- When going down a hill in a wheelie, a spotter cannot help you balance without disturbing your balance. In this case the spotter can only walk to your side and be ready to keep you from falling forward if you land on all four wheels or be ready to catch you should you begin to tip back to the rear. You will need to communicate to your spotter which method of spotting you prefer since it will generally not be possible for the spotter to do both.

- If a spotter is helping you learn this new skill, use a spotter strap as described and explained in Section 1.9 Wheelies.

How an assistant can help

To help you get a feel for what it will be like to go down a ramp in a wheelie, an assistant can fully assist you by balancing you in a wheelie and taking you down a ramp as follows:

- With your assistant holding onto your push handles or supporting the back support posts with the pull straps, pop into a wheelie position.
- Maintaining the wheelie position, roll forward onto the ramp. Your assistant will hold onto the push handles.
- Your assistant can pull back on the push handles to reduce your speed. Be sure your assistant uses leg rather than back strength. (See Section 5.1 for more information about how to prevent injuries.)
- Apply pressure on the handrims to help reduce your speed.
- When you are on level ground, ask your assistant to lower your wheelchair casters back to the ground out of the wheelie position.
- Note that if the ramp is too steep for you to go down in a wheelie on your own, that it is generally safer to have your assistant get behind you and go down the ramp backwards.

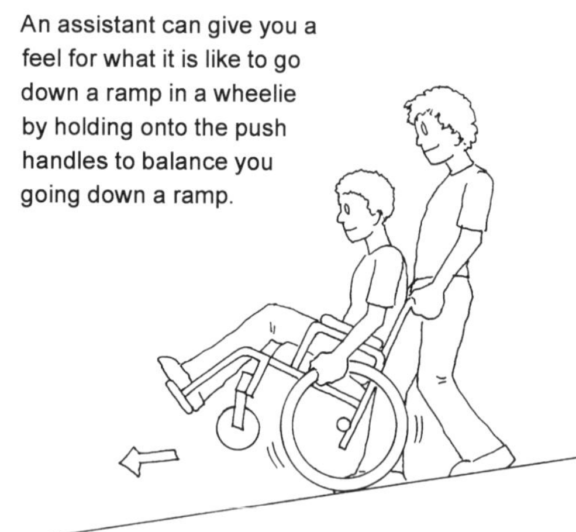

An assistant can give you a feel for what it is like to go down a ramp in a wheelie by holding onto the push handles to balance you going down a ramp.

Zigzagging down forward

Zigzagging is a way to descend very steep ramps facing forward while maintaining control. While zigzagging can decrease the steepness of the slope you experience, it will also increase the amount of side slope you must cope with. Side slopes are addressed later in Section 2.6.

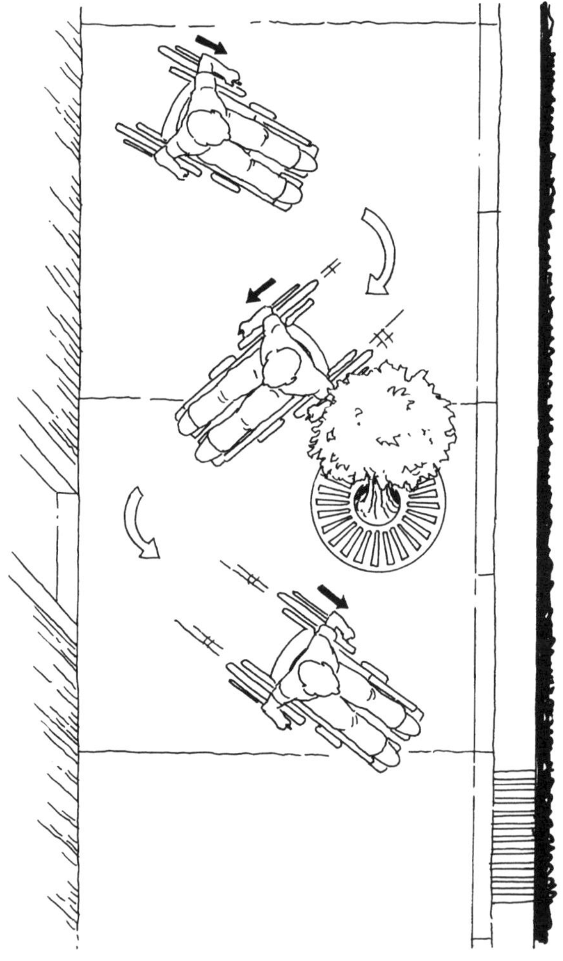

Zig-zagging down a ramp can help slow you down enough to maintain control.

- Travel down the ramp in a "Z" pattern. The more you angle your wheelchair, the greater the side slope you will have to travel across.
- Grip mostly with your uphill hand. This will prevent your wheelchair from heading straight down the ramp.
- Zigzagging down a ramp can help slow you down enough to maintain control.
- To turn, grip with your downhill hand.
- This can also be done in a wheelie.
- You can also help reduce your speed by applying more pressure on the handrims. Less pressure on the handrims will increase your speed.
- If you do this too fast or if the slope is too steep, you will tip over to the side.

How a spotter can help

- Walk on the downhill side of the wheelchair user.
- Prevent the wheelchair user from tipping sideways.
- Be sure to stay out of the wheelchair user's path of travel.

Going down a ramp backward

Using one handrail

- Examine the ramp for obstacles.
- Turn your wheelchair until your back is to the ramp.
- Grasp the handrail with one hand. With the other hand, grip your wheelchair's tire or handrim in a forward position.
- Lean forward (toward the top of the hill) to bring your center of gravity forward making you and your wheelchair more stable.
- Start sliding down the ramp backward, squeezing one handrim and holding onto the handrail with your other hand to slow your progress.

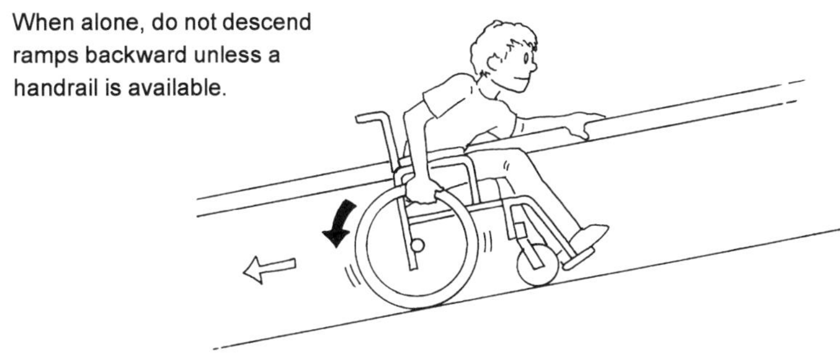
When alone, do not descend ramps backward unless a handrail is available.

How to ask for assistance

- Examine the ramp for obstacles.
- Turn until your back is to the ramp.
- Have your assistant step behind your wheelchair and grasp the push handles or back support posts with the pull straps.
- Lean forward to bring your center of gravity forward, making you and your wheelchair more stable.
- Your assistant can pull on the push handles or back support posts with the pull straps to initiate the descent. Be sure your assistant uses leg strength rather than back strength to slow your descent. (See Section 5.1 for more information on how to prevent back injuries.)
- As your assistant begins to back down the ramp, shift your weight further forward and apply pressure on the handrims in a forward position to help brake or hold onto one handrail and apply pressure to the handrim with the other hand.

How a spotter can help

- Position yourself behind the wheelchair user.
- Prevent the wheelchair user from descending the ramp too quickly.

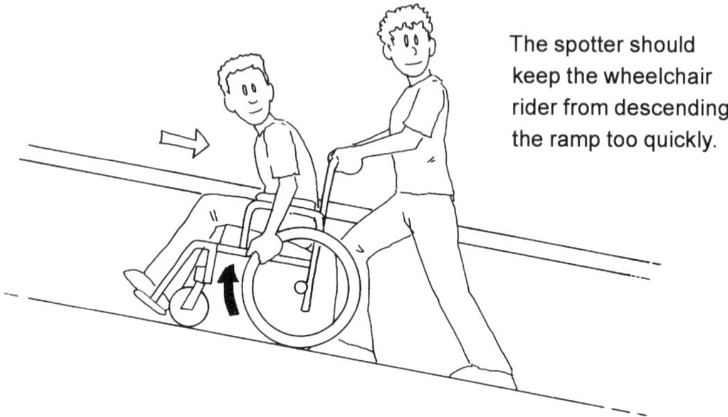

The spotter should keep the wheelchair rider from descending the ramp too quickly.

Helpful Hint

Slowing your wheels down with your hands may give you "hot hands." Avoid this discomfort by wearing gloves or stopping to rest on the way down a ramp.

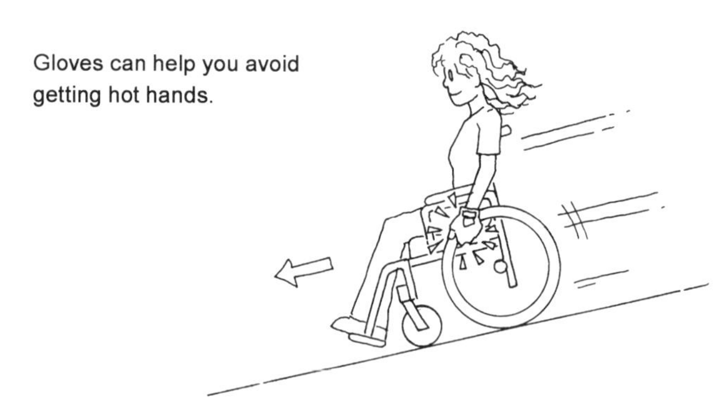

Gloves can help you avoid getting hot hands.

Resting on a Ramp

The safest way to rest on a ramp is to wait until you reach a level landing. Otherwise, your wheelchair might tip sideways while pivoting on a side slope. Techniques for crossing side slopes are found in Section 2.6.

You may need to turn sideways to rest while traveling on a ramp or need to change propulsion directions to alternate using your pulling and pushing muscles.

Turning on a ramp / Propelling up a ramp backward

With a little practice, you can turn around safely on the incline of most, but not all, ramps. Always keep your weight shifted uphill when turning around on a ramp, as this will help prevent your wheelchair from tipping over. Some people propel as far forward up a ramp as they can, then turn around and pull themselves up the ramp backward the rest of the way. Others can use their feet to propel themselves backward up a ramp. This technique will not work for someone who does not have lower back muscles.

- Propel forward up the ramp.
- When you need to give your pushing muscles a break, turn your wheelchair around by pulling on one handrim and pushing on the other.
- To avoid tipping over, lean into the hill as you turn.
- Lean back into the hill when you are facing downhill.
- Now propel your wheelchair up the ramp, by pulling backward on the handrims.
- When you reach the top, check behind you for any oncoming traffic before turning around and proceeding forward.

Section 2.6

Side Slopes

A side slope is the side-to-side slant of a walkway. Sidewalks are built with side slopes to permit rainwater to flow off the curb and into the gutter instead of pooling on the path or flooding buildings. Standard walkways should have side slopes no steeper than 2%. Steeper side slopes occur in many places, including curb ramps and when crossing a ramp or driveway crossing sideways. Side slopes also occur whenever you propel across a hill at an angle rather than straight up and down. Outdoor recreation trails can also have significant side slopes.

The experience of moving on walkways with side slopes will be different for everyone, depending on your trunk stability, tire tread, the type of surface, and the type of wheelchair. Your wheelchair will tend to turn in the direction of the slope, and you will have to compensate by gripping or dragging the uphill hand and pushing with the downhill hand. Steep side slopes might cause your wheelchair to tip. Remember to lean into the hill to avoid tipping over.

Before practicing the skills in this section, you should be able to propel a wheelchair forward and backward and remain seated when your balance is challenged.

Traveling on a Side Slope

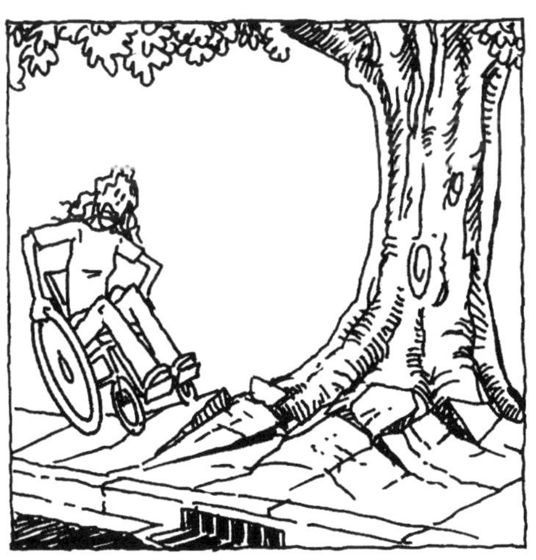

With a spotter, find a side slope that will challenge your balance from side-to-side. You can practice this by propelling across wide, steep ramps or driveways. Ask your spotter to walk on your downward side to prevent you from losing your balance.

- Maintain your balance by leaning into the hill.
- Keep your wheelchair centered on the walkway. This way you will have room to correct yourself if you start to slip downhill. You will also have more room to move around obstacles in the uphill direction.
- As your caster wheels veer downhill, push your wheelchair with the hand on the downhill side and drag your uphill hand forward on the handrim to keep your wheelchair moving in a straight line.
- Lean uphill to avoid tipping over.

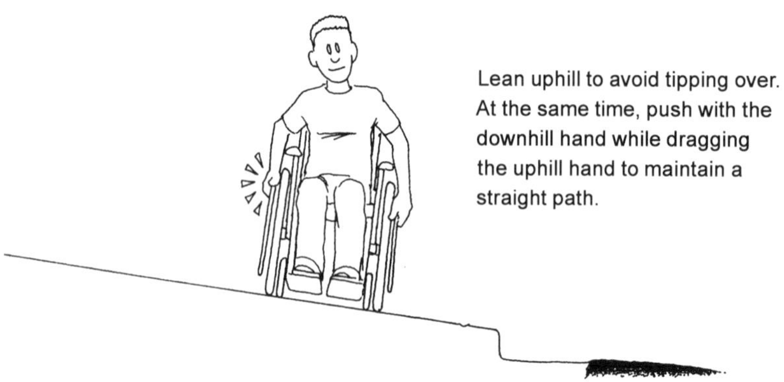

How to ask for assistance

If a side slope is too severe for you to cross safely, try to find an alternative route. If you cannot find an alternate route, ask someone for assistance.

- Tell the assistant that your wheelchair will tend to turn and roll in the direction of the downhill slope. Ask the assistant to hold onto your push handles or back support and to assist you with maintaining a straight path of travel across the side slope.
- If you have a climbing sling or a piece of rope or webbing, you can attach it near the top of the front caster on the frame of your wheelchair on the uphill side of your wheelchair. You can ask your assistant to pull up and forward. This will prevent your wheelchair from veering in the downhill direction of the side slope. This is particularly useful on outdoor recreation hiking trails that may have more substantial side slopes.

How a spotter can help

- Walk on the downhill side of the wheelchair user.
- Be ready to keep the wheelchair rolling in a straight path and prevent it from tipping over sideways.

Section 2.7

Curb Ramps

Curb ramps are designed to provide a more accessible path of travel between the sidewalk and the street. Unfortunately, curb ramps can be dangerous and have been the site of many accidents involving people using wheelchairs. Always proceed with caution when crossing a street at curb ramps. Street crossings are where many pedestrians are injured as a result of conflicts with motor vehicles. As a wheelchair user you are not immune from this hazard.

Even if the curb is ramped at the standard 1:12 slope, there is often a much steeper slope and/or small lip where the curb ramp reaches the gutter and the street. There is also a dip where the curb ramp meets the gutter which goes back uphill to meet the asphalt in the street.

Approach curb ramps slowly. If there is any interference with the foot supports or the anti-tip devices, you will stop abruptly and may be thrown from your wheelchair. It is important to have sufficient foot support clearance at curb ramps as there is often a small step transition where the curb ramp meets the gutter.

Before practicing the techniques in this section, you should be able to propel your wheelchair forward and backward and be capable of maintaining your balance when it is challenged. You need to be able to travel up and down a ramp. Knowing how to pop a partial and/or full wheelie will give you more options when encountering curb ramps. Practice on different types of curb ramps with a spotter to determine what ramps you are able to ascend and descend safely. If you do not feel comfortable using a particular curb ramp/gutter combination independently, ask for assistance.

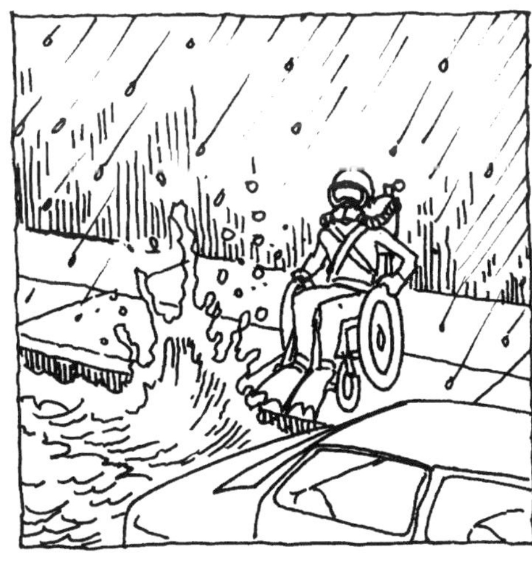

With care, you can avoid catching your casters or footrests and falling where the downslope of the curb ramp meets the up-slope of the gutter and street.

Going Down a Curb Ramp

Always travel in the center of curb ramps. The flared sides of a curb ramp have a slope and a side slope. In combination, they can easily tilt you off balance. If the curb ramp projects out into the street, be aware of the flare slopes on either side.

Descending forward

On four wheels

You may be able to descend gradual curb ramps by heading straight down on four wheels.

- Check the sidewalk, curb ramp, gutter, and street for cracks, lips, and uneven surfaces. Be aware of traffic and other pedestrians.
- Head down the center of the curb ramp.
- Just like when you roll down a standard ramp, lean back to avoid falling forward.

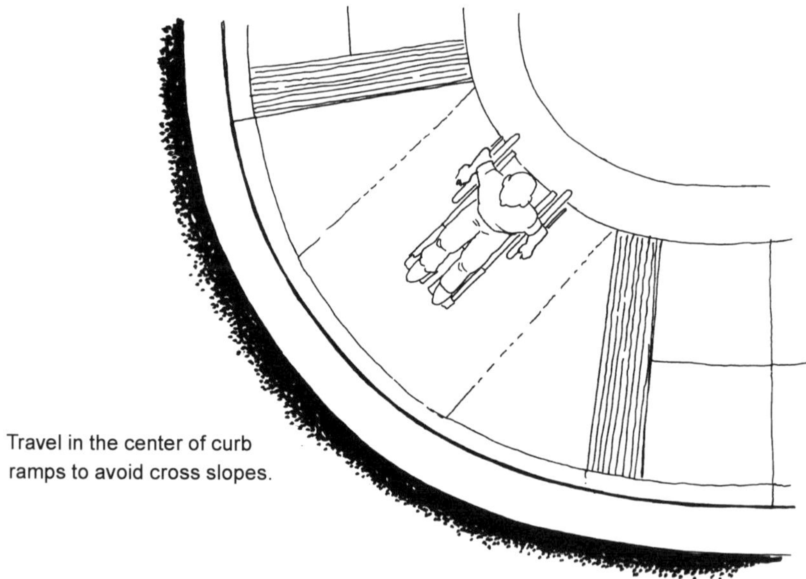

Travel in the center of curb ramps to avoid cross slopes.

- Grip your handrims to slow your wheelchair down.
- As you reach the bottom, you may need to pop a partial wheelie to roll over a lip at the gutter.
- Wait until you reach level ground before turning left or right.

In a wheelie

It is often desirable to descend a steep curb ramp in a wheelie to avoid falling forward out of your wheelchair. It also prevents you from catching your caster wheels on uneven surfaces.

- Check the sidewalk, curb ramp, and street for cracks, lips, and uneven surfaces. Be aware of traffic and pedestrians.
- Head down the center of the curb ramp.
- While still on a level surface, pop a wheelie.
- Maintaining the wheelie position, descend the curb ramp slowly. Applying greater pressure to the handrims will slow you down.
- Wait until your rear wheels have reached the gutter before coming out of the wheelie position.

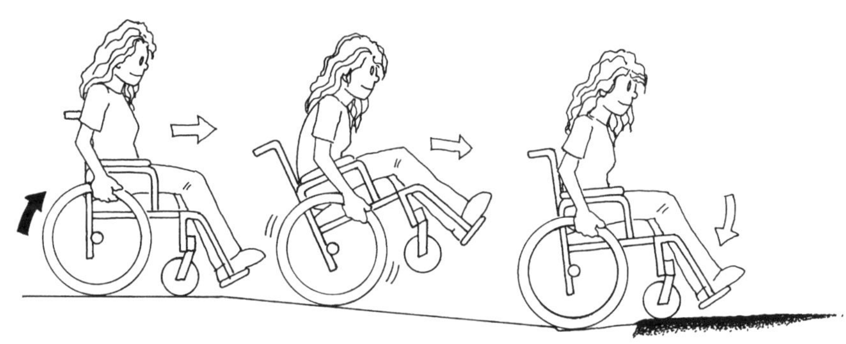

1. Pop a wheelie at the top of the curb ramp.
2. Descend the ramp in a wheelie.
3. Come down out of the wheelie only after your back wheels have reached the transition between the bottom of the curb ramp and the gutter.

How to ask for assistance

If a curb ramp is steep or there are obstacles you do not feel comfortable crossing independently, ask for assistance.

- Have an assistant hold the push handles or back support posts with the pull straps on your wheelchair.
- Have an assistant back you down the curb ramp backwards (see Descending backward just ahead in the text) and then turn around at the gutter or…
- With your assistant, tip your wheelchair into a wheelie.
- Maintaining the wheelie position, slowly descend the curb ramp.
- The assistant can help slow the descent by pulling back on the push handles or back support posts with the pull straps. You can help slow your descent by applying pressure to the handrims.
- After reaching the bottom of the curb ramp, ask your assistant to lower your wheelchair out of the wheelie position.

How a spotter can help when going down a curb ramp on four wheels

- Remain in front and to the side of the wheelchair user.
- Prevent the wheelchair user from toppling forward out of the chair.
- Be sure to stay out of the wheelchair user's path of travel.
- Have the wheelchair user wear his or her lap belt.
- Stand behind the wheelchair user with your hands close to the push handles or back support posts with pull straps.
- Prevent the wheelchair from tipping over.
- At the bottom of the curb ramp, the front caster wheels or footplates could hit the gutter slope or catch in a grate and launch the rider forward out of the wheelchair. To avoid this, the spotter can place a hand on the rider's shoulder to prevent a forward fall at the base of the curb ramp.

How a spotter can help when going down a curb ramp in a wheelie

- Stand behind the wheelchair user with your hands close to the push handles or back support posts with the pull straps.
- If the wheelchair user is just learning this new skill, use a spotter strap as described and explained in Section 1.9 Wheelies.

Descending backward

If the curb ramp is steep, there are surface irregularities at the base, or there is a sharp incline back up into the street, it might be easier for you to descend backwards.

- Check the sidewalk, curb ramp, and street for uneven surfaces. Be aware of street traffic and other pedestrians.
- Examine how steep the curb ramp is, where the side slopes are, and what the terrain at the curb ramp base is like.
- Turn to back down the curb ramp.
- As you descend the curb ramp, lean forward to avoid tipping over backward.
- Grip the handrims to slow the rolling motion.
- Continue rolling backward until you clear any surface irregularities. Then turn around and proceed facing forward.

How to ask for assistance

- Turn your wheelchair so your back is to the curb ramp.
- Have your assistant stand behind your wheelchair, with his or her back to the curb ramp. Ask your assistant to hold your

wheelchair's push handles or back support posts with the pull straps.

- Together with your assistant, back down the curb ramp.
- Your assistant can slow the descent by pushing forward on the push handles or frame. You can help slow the descent by applying pressure to the handrims.

How a spotter can help

- Stand behind the wheelchair with your hands close to the push handles or back support posts with the pull straps.
- Have the wheelchair user lean forward to prevent the wheelchair from tipping back as he or she rolls down the curb ramp.
- Make sure the wheelchair doesn't roll too quickly. Watch for anti-tip device clearance at the base of the curb ramp.
- If the wheelchair user is just learning this new skill, use a spotter strap as described and explained in Section 1.9 Wheelies.
- Watch for oncoming traffic.

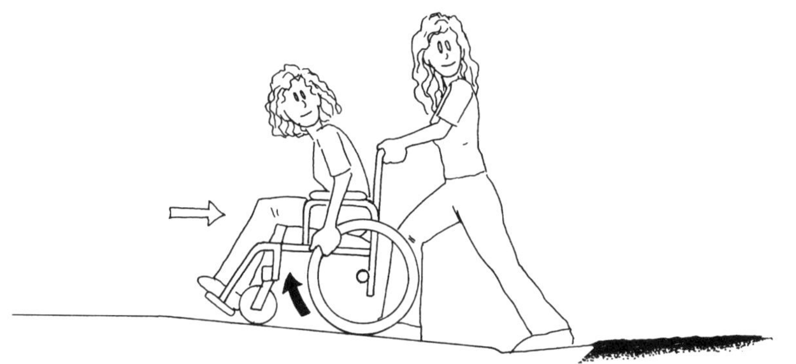

An assistant can help slow a backward curb ramp descent.

Going Up a Curb Ramp

Practice ascending different types of curb ramps with a spotter to determine what angle of ascent you can safely handle. With a spotter, climb increasingly steeper curb ramps until you reach a point where the front caster wheels start lifting off the ground. This is beyond the steepest curb ramp you can climb without tipping your wheelchair over backward. To avoid this, ask a spotter to hold onto the push handles or back support posts with the pull straps to keep your wheels grounded. A spotter can also provide extra pushing power.

Approach the curb ramp so you are headed straight up the center of it into the sidewalk. The flared sides have a slope and a side slope that can be dangerous to negotiate. If the curb ramp projects out into the street, be aware of the flared slopes on each side.

Going up forward

On four wheels

- Pop a partial wheelie if you need extra clearance for the foot supports at the street/curb ramp transition.
- Lean forward as you propel up the curb ramp to prevent your wheelchair from tipping over backward.
- Wait until you have reached the level landing above the curb ramp before changing your direction of travel.

How to ask for assistance

- Ask your assistant to push you up the curb ramp using the push handles or back support posts with the pull straps.
- Push forward on the handrims and/or tires at the same time.

How a spotter can help

- Stand behind the wheelchair user with your hands close to the push handles or back support posts with the pull straps.
- Keep the wheelchair user from tipping over backward.
- If the wheelchair user is just learning this new skill, use a spotter strap as described and explained in Section 1.9 Wheelies.

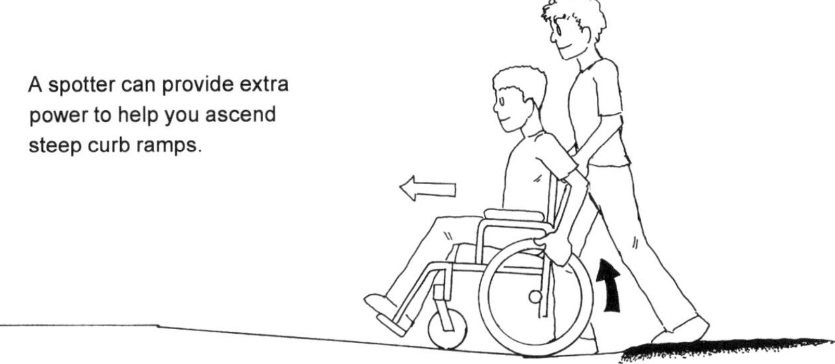
A spotter can provide extra power to help you ascend steep curb ramps.

Going up backward

Climb the curb ramp backward if your pulling muscles are stronger. This is also easier for people who propel their wheelchairs with their feet.

- Examine the transition from the street to the curb ramp. Check for cracks, lips, and uneven surfaces. Be aware of traffic and pedestrians in the street and on the sidewalk.
- When you reach the curb ramp, turn your wheelchair around. Make sure you are aimed toward the center of the curb ramp into the sidewalk. The flared sides have a slope and a side slope that can tip you over. If a curb ramp projects out into the street, it may have flares sloping out on each side.
- Propel backward to ascend the curb ramp, leaning against the back support to avoid falling forward.
- Wait until you have reached the level landing at the top of the curb ramp before turning around and continuing on your way.

How to ask for assistance

- If you need assistance, ascend the curb ramp going forward.
- Ask your assistant to push you forward up the curb ramp using the push handles or back support posts with the pull straps.
- Push forward on the handrims at the same time.

How a spotter can help you going up backward

- Stand to the side facing the wheelchair user.
- Follow the wheelchair user up the curb ramp and prevent him or her from falling forward by placing a hand on his or her shoulder.

Section 2.8

Curbs

Curbs are the transition point between sidewalks and streets. If curb ramps are missing, in poor repair, or blocked, you will have to go up or down the curb. The lower the curb, the easier it is to negotiate. With practice, you may be able to go up and down fairly high curbs.

To go up and down curbs, you must be able to propel your wheelchair forward and backward. You will be able to perform more of the curb techniques in this chapter if you can pop a partial and/or full wheelie, move forward in the wheelie position, and maintain a sitting position when your balance is challenged.

The skills in this section require a significant amount of wheelchair experience and strength to accomplish, and may expose you, and any assistants helping you, to physical strain and serious injury. By performing these techniques, you must recognize the danger inherent in these actions and execute them with caution knowing that you are taking a risk.

When learning the techniques in this chapter, use curbs in quiet areas, and avoid busy streets. Practice with a spotter until you can safely and consistently go up and down curbs. Climb increasingly higher curbs with a spotter to determine the highest you can handle independently.

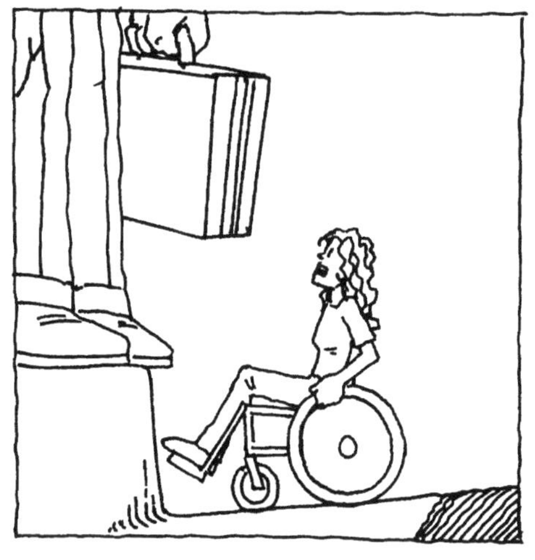

Going Up Curbs

If you are unable to pop a full or partial wheelie while moving forward, practice initiating them as you move over lines in the sidewalk. This exercise will help you perfect your wheelie timing before you attempt to climb a curb.

Your foot support clearance may affect your ability to ascend and descend curbs, especially if you cannot perform a wheelie. Avoid hitting your foot supports on the edge of the curb, as you could fall forward. Large rubber or pneumatic caster wheels will roll over curb edges more easily than small plastic ones.

Ascending forward

Rolling

Depending on your strength, you can simply roll over curbs less than two inches high.

- Roll your front caster wheels against the curb. (This is easiest when the casters are in the rear trailing position.)
- Pushing on the handrims, move the caster wheels onto the curb.
- Reach back and grab the handrims.
- Leaning forward, push until the rear wheels are on the curb.

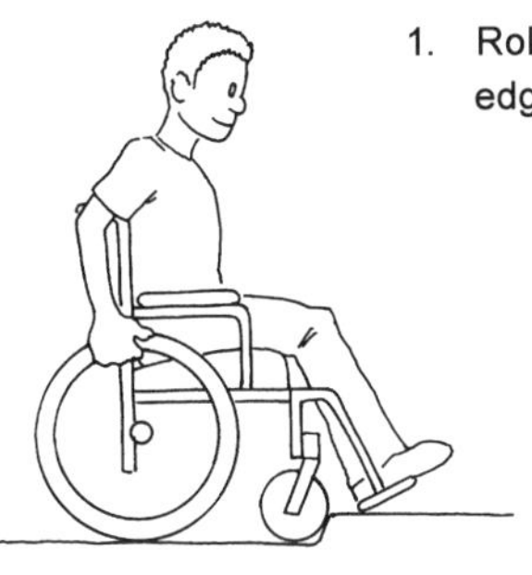

1. Roll up to the edge of the curb.

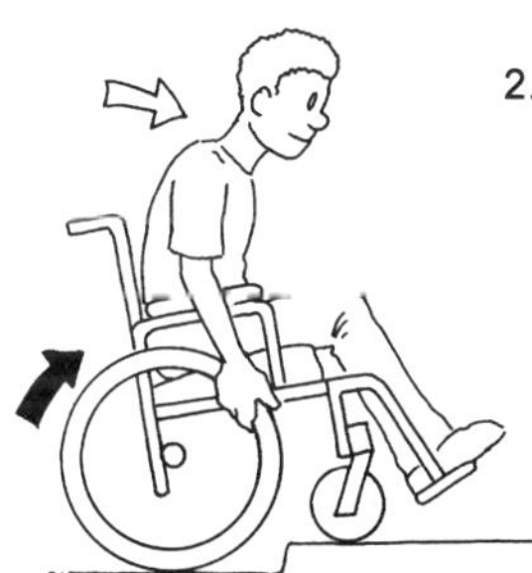

2. Push forward to roll the caster wheels up onto the curb while leaning forward.

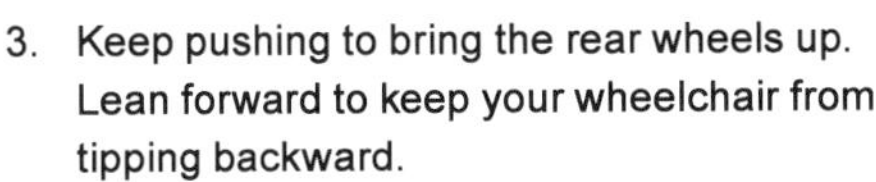

3. Keep pushing to bring the rear wheels up. Lean forward to keep your wheelchair from tipping backward.

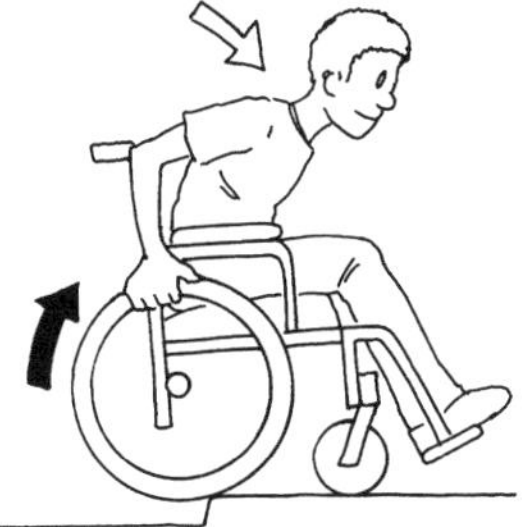

Popping a partial wheelie

- Facing the curb, pop a wheelie.
- Move forward in the wheelie until the caster wheels are past the curb.
- Leaning forward, continue propelling your wheelchair up onto the curb by forcefully pushing on the handrims.

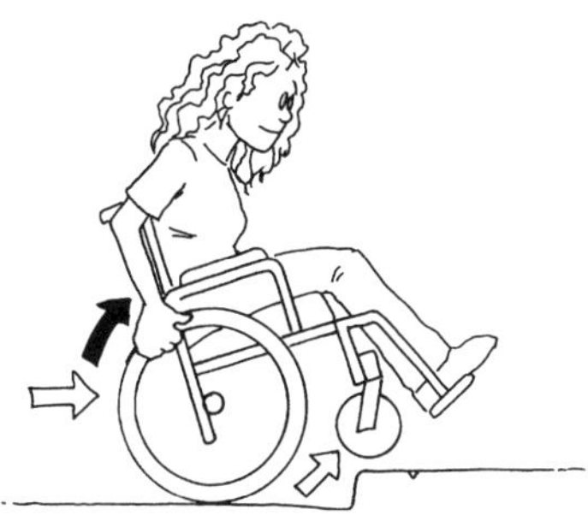

1. Pop a wheelie as you approach the curb. Roll in the wheelie until your rear wheels contact the curb and your front wheels are on the curb.

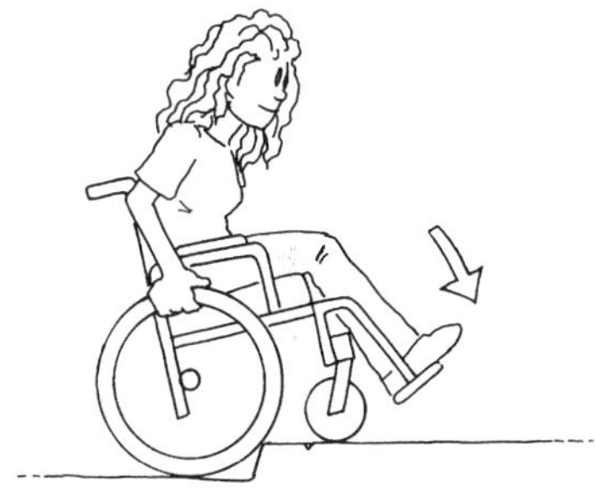

2. As your casters come down on the top of the curb, lean forward while continuing to push. This will start to put the rear wheels up onto the curb.

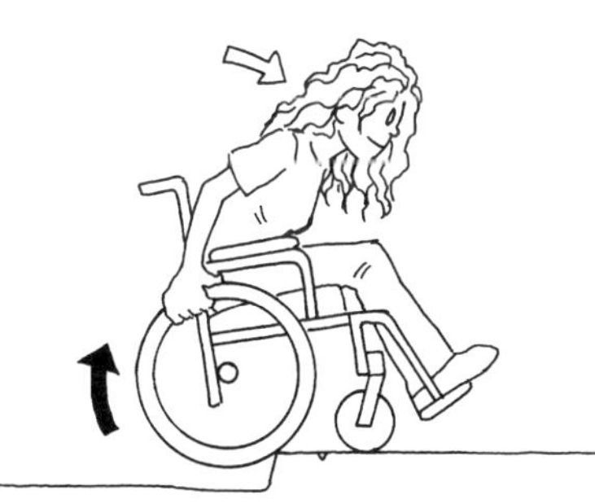

3. Lean forward as you push on the handrims.

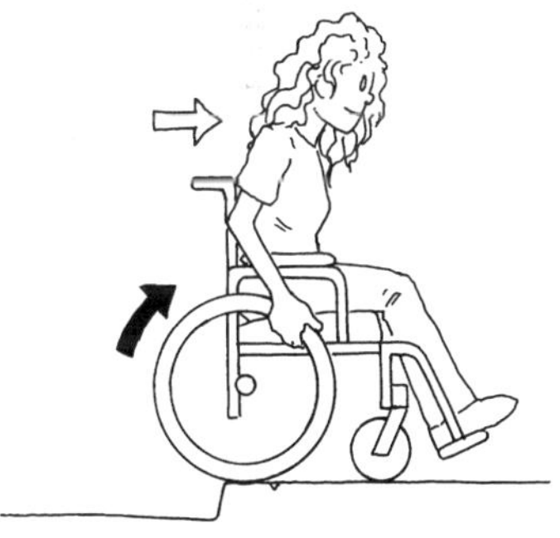

4. Continue pushing, bringing your rear wheels up onto the curb.

Using momentum and popping a partial wheelie

- Approach the curb with some speed, gathering momentum.
- When you are almost at the curb, pop a partial wheelie and continue moving forward, letting the caster wheels down onto the top of the curb. Popping the partial wheelie too early may cause you to fall out of the wheelie before reaching the curb, while popping it too late may cause you to hit the face of the curb edge and you may fall forward.
- When the front caster wheels are on the curb, propel the large rear wheels up by reaching back and pushing firmly on the handrims. Leaning forward as you ascend the curb will help you keep the momentum going forward and up the curb.

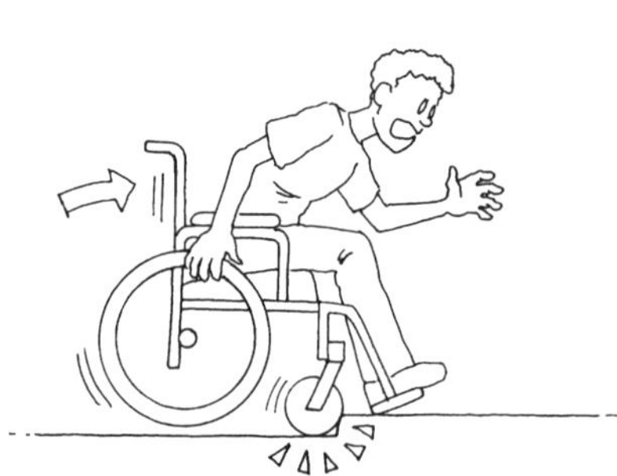

Popping the wheelie too early or too late may cause your casters to hit the curb, pitching you forward.

Pulling on stationary objects

You can also use a parking meter, sign, or other well anchored post to pull yourself up.

- Roll your wheelchair forward until the front caster wheels rest against the curb. The parking meter or post should be forward and just off to one side of your chair.
- Push firmly on the handrims to pop a wheelie and get the front caster wheels on top of the curb. If this causes you to exceed your balance point, quickly grip the pole with the nearest hand.
- Reach forward and grasp the pole with the nearest hand. Tug to make sure the pole is firmly anchored.
- With your other hand, push firmly on the handrim while pulling on the pole until your rear wheels are up on the curb.

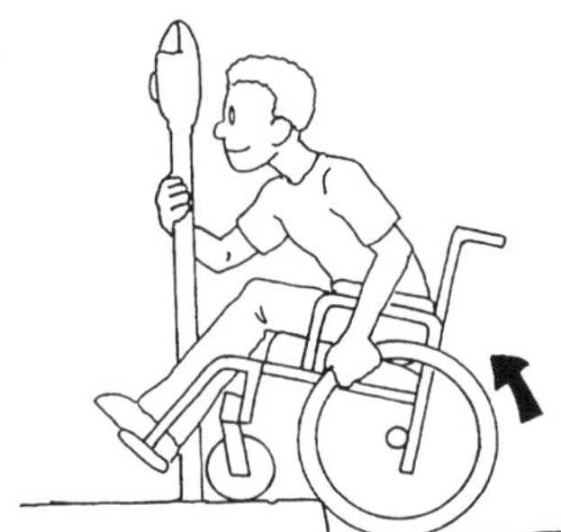

You can use parking meters, street signs, or other solidly anchored poles to help pull yourself up curbs.

How a spotter can help

- Position yourself behind the wheelchair user and place your hands near the push handles or on the back support posts with the pull straps.
- This is a good situation to use a spotting strap placed around the X-cross frame of a folding chair or the axle bar of a rigid chair as described and explained in Section 1.9 Wheelies.
- Keep the spotting strap loose while the person is moving into a wheelie and over the curb, while in a position to pull the spotting strap tight if the person begins to fall backwards.
- Try not to influence the balance of the wheelchair, but be ready to assist the rider if necessary.
- Prevent the wheelchair from tipping backward.
- Keep one hand near the rider's shoulder to prevent a forward fall if he or she pops the wheelie too soon.
- Provide side-to-side support if the wheelchair tips to one side.

How to ask for assistance

Getting pulled

If you can get the front caster wheels up onto the curb but do not have enough strength to push the rear wheels up on the curb, an assistant can help pull you onto the curb. This technique is useful on small curbs that do not require exceptional effort to climb.

- Have the assistant stand on the curb sideways facing you.
- Grasp one of your assistant's wrists, right to right or left to left.
- Grip your wheelchair frame with your free hand to avoid being pulled out of the chair.
- On your count of three, have your assistant pull you forward smoothly so as not to jerk you out of the seat of your wheelchair, until all four wheels are safely on the curb. Your assistant should use leg strength and body weight rather than back strength to pull. (See Section 5.1 for more information about preventing injuries.)

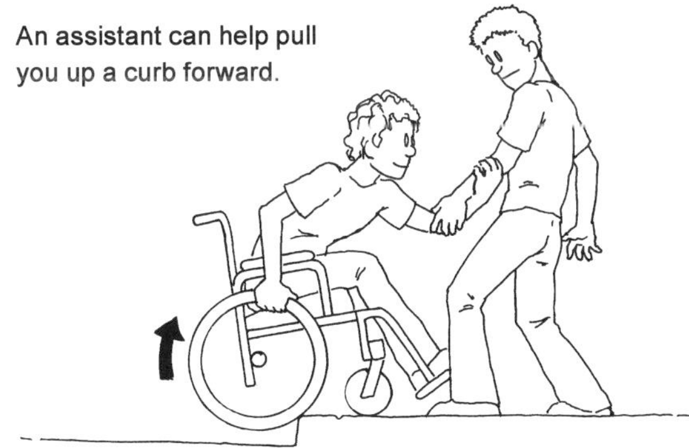

An assistant can help pull you up a curb forward.

- If you have a climbing sling or a piece of rope or webbing, you can attach it near the top of the front caster on the frame of your wheelchair and have your assistant pull up and forward on the sling to pull you up the curb. You should lean forward and push forward on the handrims while your assistant pulls forward on the sling or strap. With a climbing sling or strap on each side of your wheelchair, you can have two assistants help you up a large curb.

Getting pushed

If you do not have enough strength to climb the curb alone, you can also have an assistant help push you up.

- Roll forward until both front caster wheels rest against the curb.
- Ask your assistant to stand sideways behind your wheelchair. Have him or her push a hip into the back of the chair while pushing down on a push handle or back post. At the same time, you should pop a partial wheelie and push forward on the handrims to move your caster wheels onto the curb. To avoid back injuries the spotter should not twist at the waist. (See Section 5.1 for more information about preventing injuries.)
- Together with your assistant, push forward a second time until the rear wheels are on the curb.

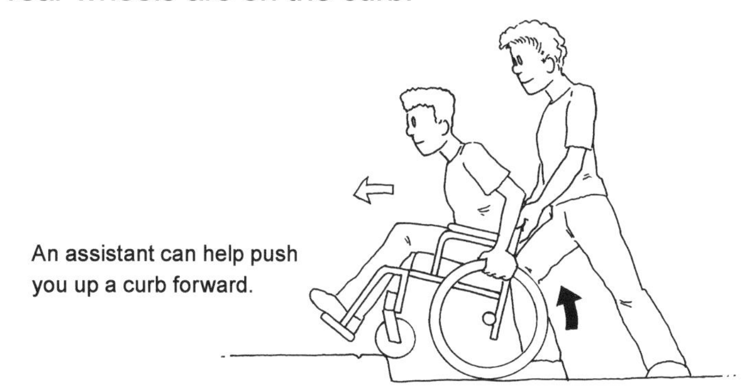

An assistant can help push you up a curb forward.

Ascending backward with assistance

- Roll backward until the rear wheels are against the curb.
- Have an assistant on the curb place one foot between the rear wheels and the other on the sidewalk.
- This technique is easiest when you start in a wheelie position. After you have your assistant tip you back into a wheelie, on your count of three, have the assistant pull up and back using leg strength and body weight while you pull on the rear wheels. This will pull your wheelchair up onto the curb.
- Once on the sidewalk and clear of the curb, you can lower the front caster wheels onto the sidewalk by holding your wheels still and asking your assistant to lower the front wheels to the ground.

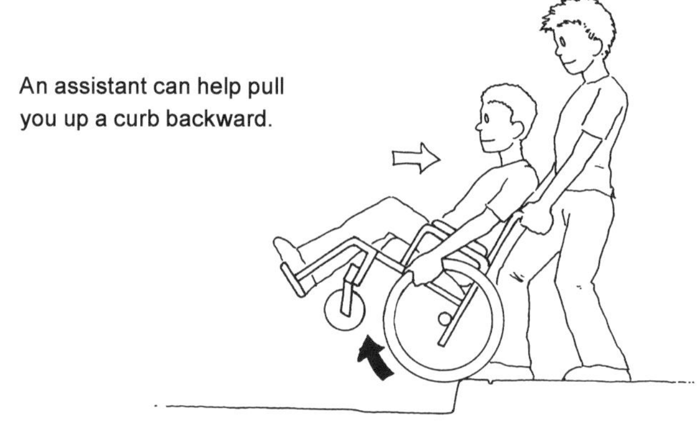

An assistant can help pull you up a curb backward.

Going Down Curbs

Descending forward

- Facing the curb, pop a wheelie.
- Move forward in the wheelie position until the rear wheels are at the edge of the curb.
- Lean forward slightly as you are going off the edge of the curb so that the rear wheels land first and the caster wheels land at the same time or just after the rear wheels. If your casters land first, your wheelchair may tip forward.

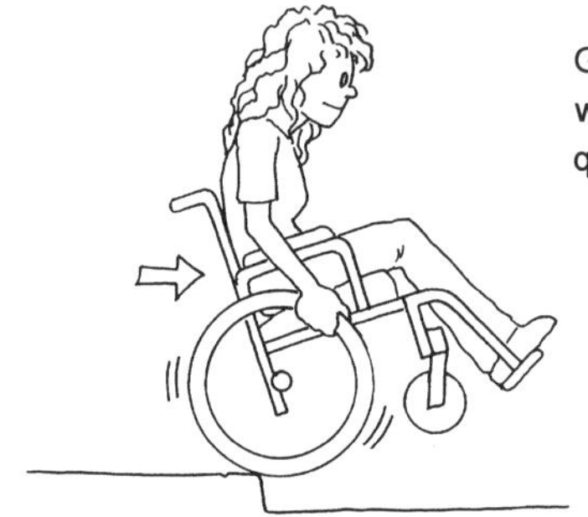

Going down a curb forward and in a wheelie can be the smoothest and quickest way to reach the street.

How a spotter can help

- Stand behind the wheelchair user and place your hands close to the push handles or back support posts with the pull straps. This is a good place to use a spotting strap placed around the X-cross frame of a folding chair or the axle bar of a rigid chair. The general use of a spotter strap is described and explained in Section 1.9 Wheelies.
- Keep the spotting strap loose while the person is moving into a wheelie and over the curb, while in a position to pull the spotting strap tight if the person is falling backwards.
- Try not to influence the balance of the wheelchair, but be ready to assist the rider if necessary.
- Prevent the wheelchair user from falling over backward.
- Provide side-to-side support if one rear wheel leaves the curb before the other and the wheelchair tips to one side.
- Make sure the wheelchair remains in the wheelie until the curb is descended.

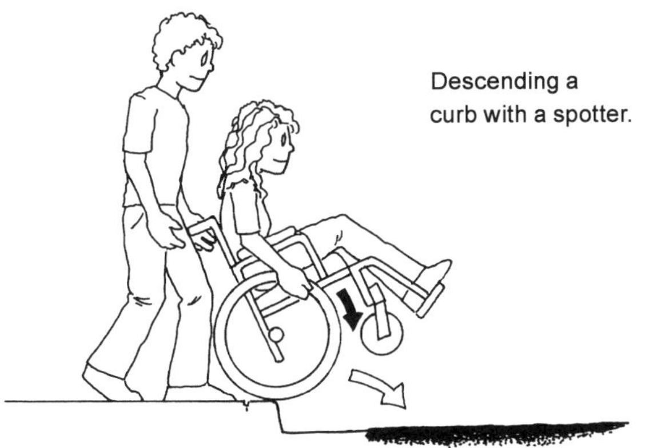

Descending a curb with a spotter.

How to ask for assistance

If the curb is too high for you to safely perform the above maneuver, ask an assistant to help.

- Ask your assistant to stand behind you, holding the push handles.
- Roll forward toward the curb.
- When your casters are on the edge, ask your assistant to hold onto the push handles or back support posts with the pull straps of your wheelchair.
- Have your assistant tip you into a wheelie and roll you forward as you propel down the curb. Ask him/her to do this slowly so you don't crash down the curb too forcefully.

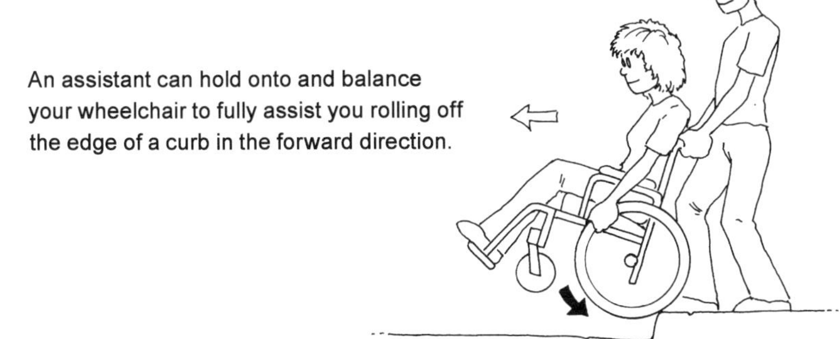

An assistant can hold onto and balance your wheelchair to fully assist you rolling off the edge of a curb in the forward direction.

Descending backward

If you cannot pop, maintain, and maneuver in a wheelie well, you might find it easier to descend a curb backwards. If descending a curb traveling backward, avoid hitting your foot supports on the way down.

- Roll backward until the rear wheels are at the curb edge.
- Lean forward and reach far forward on the handrims.
- Slowly move backward by pulling on the handrims until your rear wheels drop onto the street. Your caster wheels should still be resting on the curb.
- Slowly sit upright as you reverse and pivot to face the street, keeping your wheelchair in a wheelie as much as you can.
- Lower yourself out of the wheelie and continue on your way.

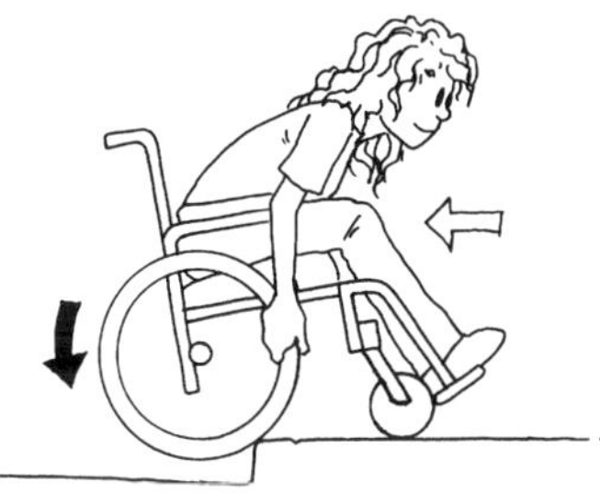

Leaning far forward as you back down the curb will help prevent you from tipping over backward.

Warning: If the curb's height exceeds your balance point, you could fall over backward during this maneuver. With a new curb, always practice this first with a spotter since it is difficult to determine the exact height of a curb from up on the sidewalk. If the curb is too high and you do this without a spotter you will tip over backward as soon as your rear wheels contact the gutter.

How a spotter can help

- Stand behind the wheelchair user.
- Catch the rider if he or she starts to fall back or to the side.
- If the wheelchair user is just learning this new skill, use a spotter strap as described and explained in Section 1.9 Wheelies.

How to ask for assistance

- Roll backward toward the curb.
- When your rear wheels are on the edge, ask your assistant to hold onto the push handles.
- As you slowly roll backward, ask the assistant to turn a hip into the back of the chair. Make sure the assistant does not twist at the waist, but instead stands sideways with her or his entire body.
- With a hip braced against the back of the chair, the assistant should take small steps backward as you roll backward, easing your wheelchair to the ground.
- You may want to ask the assistant to push down on the push handles as you bring your caster wheels off the curb so they do not drop to the ground too quickly.
- Ask the assistant not to release your wheelchair until all four wheels are in contact with the ground.

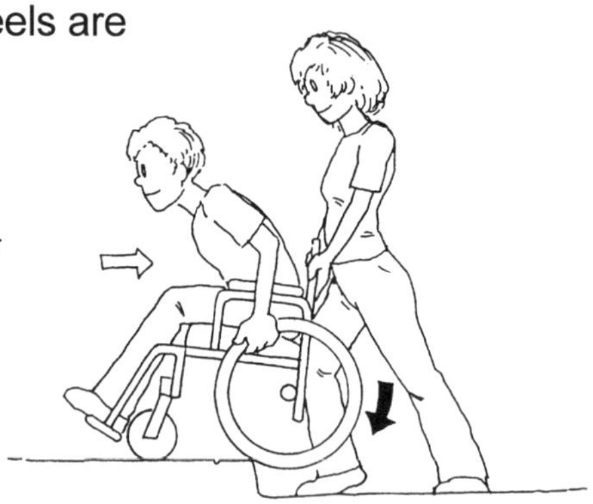

An assistant can help lower you down a curb in a slow and controlled manner.

Section 2.9

Stairs

Most public buildings with stairs in the United States are also equipped with ramps, platform lifts, or elevators. However, you will probably encounter buildings where you cannot locate an accessible alternative to the stairs. In this situation, contact the building manager or other persons familiar with the facility to ask if there is an available lift or ramp; the accessible alternative to the stairs may be hidden at the building's rear or side. When a ramp, lift or elevator is not available, remind the establishment's staff that if physical access to the building is not provided, they are required to provide you with services in an accessible location. This would likely be considered a reasonable accommodation if the ownership of the building does not have the resources to install an elevator. If a spotter is helping you negotiate stairs, use a spotter strap as described and explained in Section 1.9 Wheelies.

The techniques in this section can help you ascend and descend stairs in flights, not single steps. Single or very widely spaced steps can be managed using the techniques for curbs described in Section 2.8.

Perform the techniques in this section only if you absolutely must use the stairs in an emergency and there is no other accessible alternative available. These techniques require a significant amount of wheelchair experience and strength to accomplish, and they may expose you and any assistants to physical strain and serious injury. Read the warning on page vi to learn about the risks involved in performing wheelchair skills. Falling is an unacceptable option, for some wheelchair users that may result in severe injury or death.

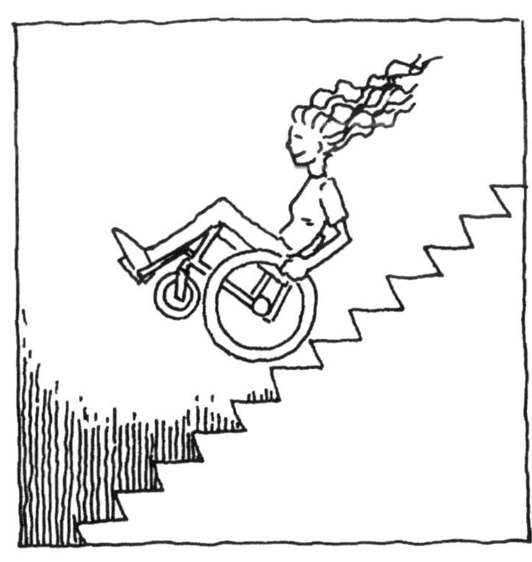

Only attempt to climb stairs alone in your wheelchair if the steps are deep enough to accommodate the full length of your wheelchair and if there is no alternative.

Before learning to perform these techniques independently, you should be able to comfortably pop a wheelie and propel yourself forward and maneuver in a wheelie position. You should also know how to climb and descend curbs using a wheelie.

When practicing these techniques, start with wide, deep stairs equipped with handrails, and attempt progressively steeper stairs until you are no longer comfortable. If the steps are too shallow to accommodate your wheels, it may be hazardous to negotiate the stairs. Practice stair techniques only if a spotter is present. Regardless of how many times you have done this, it is a good idea to have a spotter in case you have a problem.

Going Up Stairs with Assistance

Your first choice should be to climb stairs with two or three assistants.

Two assistants going up backwards

- Back up to the stairs so that your back is to the steps.
- Have one assistant stand behind your wheelchair facing the back of your wheelchair with his or her hands on the push handles or back support posts with the pull straps. Note that at the time of this publication, wheelchair manufacturers were no longer providing pull straps with wheelchairs that do not have push handles. Wheelchair manufacturers are still making upholstery with sleeves around the back support tubes. If your wheelchair has upholstery with sleeves in the upholstery you can put webbing straps through these sleeves and attach the webbing to the frame of your wheelchair and then tie or sew loops at the top of your wheelchair back support. These straps can then be used by an assistant to pull a wheelchair up steps.
- Have the assistant behind you help you tip into a wheelie.
- Have the second assistant face you and prevent you from tipping forward. This assistant should hold a portion of your wheelchair frame near your knees or feet (NOT on the removable foot supports or armrests, which can break or lift off your wheelchair easily).
- On your count of three, you will need to pull back on the handrims while the first assistant **pulls** you up onto the next step and the lower assistant **pushes** from below. Section 5.1 has information about avoiding injury while assisting a wheelchair user.

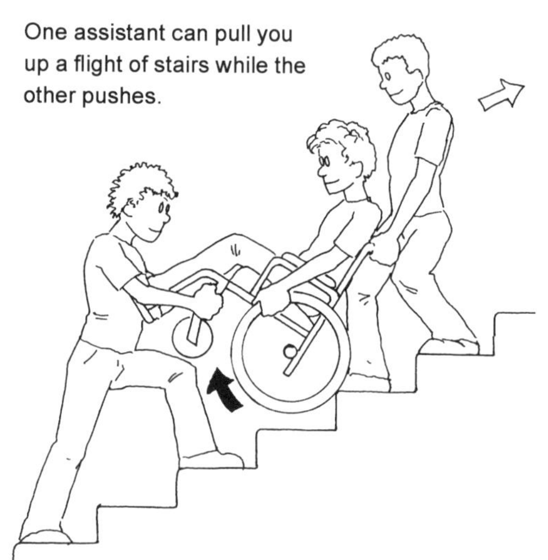
One assistant can pull you up a flight of stairs while the other pushes.

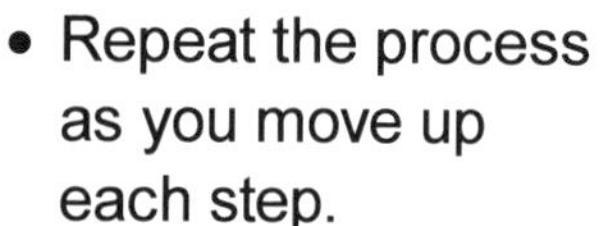

- Repeat the process as you move up each step.
- If necessary, your assistants can rest while they hold you balanced on a step.

Two or three assistants going up forwards

Some users and assistants feel that this technique is safer than two assistants going backwards.

- Position your wheelchair facing up the steps. Attach a climbing sling or a piece of rope or webbing near the top of the front caster around the frame of your wheelchair on each side of the chair.
- The two front assistants pull up and forward on each of

these straps. The rear assistant will serve as a spotter behind your wheelchair and can assist with pushing your wheelchair forward from behind by holding onto the push handles or the back support posts.

- On your count of three, the front assistants will pull up and forward on their respective pulling straps and the rear assistant will push your wheelchair forward up one step. You will pull forward on the stairway handrail and push forward on the other handrim of your wheelchair. If you can reach both stairway handrails you should pull forward on both stairway handrails.
- You should insist that your wheelchair only roll up one step at a time and that all three of the assistants step to the next step while your wheelchair rests on that particular set of steps. This allows for you to re-grip the stairway handrail and your wheelchair handrim for the next count of three.
- This technique has been used with just two assistants pulling in the front. It has also been successfully used with just one assistant pulling on one or two straps in front of the wheelchair.

One assistant

If only one assistant is available, you can either ascend the stairs backwards, or use the wheelbarrow technique.

Ascending backwards

- Together with your assistant, tip your wheelchair into a wheelie.
- Have an assistant stand behind you with hands on the push handles or back support posts with the pull straps.
- On your count of three, your assistant should pull you up to the next step while you pull back on the handrims.
- To rest, the spotter can sit down on the step above and lean the back of your wheelchair on his or her knees.
- Repeat the process as you move up each step.

Wheelbarrow technique

- Transfer out of your wheelchair and onto the floor at the foot of the stairs. Position yourself lying on your stomach or on your hands and knees.
- Have your assistant hold your feet or thighs as you raise your torso by straightening your arms.
- Climb the stairs with your arms as your assistant supports your outstretched legs.
- Another technique is to position yourself so that your back is facing the steps and your legs are stretched out in front of you. Have your assistant hold onto your feet as you slide your bottom up onto the next step one at a time. You will want to strap on a pressure relief cushion if you do not have sensation in your sitting area.
- Once you are at the top of the stairs, your assistant can carry up your wheelchair.

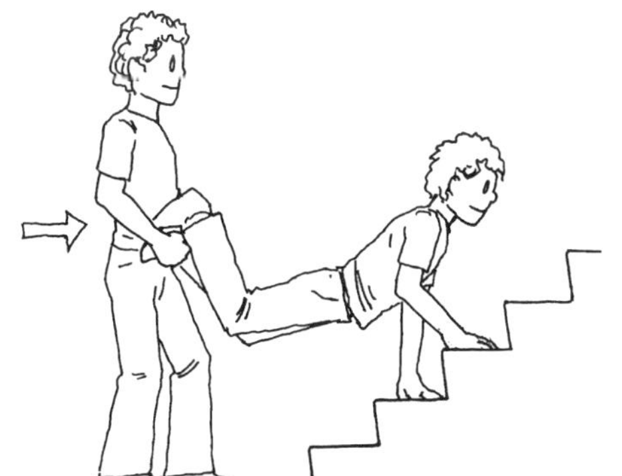

One assistant can help you climb stairs with the wheelbarrow lift.

Going Up Stairs Alone

Only climb stairs alone if you cannot find any assistants to help. Regardless of how many times you have done this, it is a good idea to have a spotter in case you have a problem.

Facing forward up the stairs

This technique should only be attempted on wide, deep steps that can accommodate the full length of your wheelchair. If the stairs are not deep enough to accommodate your wheels, you will have to climb the stairs backward without your wheelchair. If you are not wearing a lap belt during this technique, you may get pulled out of your wheelchair.

With one hand on the handrail

- Check the handrail for stability before using it. Handrails have been pulled off the wall using this technique.
- Be sure your wheelchair is square with the stairs. This will ensure that both wheels hit each step at the same time.
- When you reach the stairs, pop a partial wheelie and continue to move forward until your caster wheels are on the first step.
- Grab the handrail with the hand closest to it. Keep your other hand on the handrim.
- Lean forward, push on the handrim, and pull on the handrail at the same time to pull yourself up to the next step.
- Slide your hand farther up the handrail without letting go.
- Repeat the process one step at a time to reach the top.

With both hands on the handrail

Only attempt this technique if you are wearing a lap belt that is fastened to secure you firmly in your wheelchair.

- Check the handrail for stability before using it.
- Face the stairs squarely to ensure that both wheels hit the steps at the same time.
- As you move toward the stairs, pop a partial wheelie. Continue to move forward until your caster wheels are on the step above.
- Lean forward and grab the handrail with both hands. Be careful not to pull yourself out of your wheelchair.
- Pull yourself up to the next step. You may want to alternate using both hands on the handrail with using one hand on the handrail and pushing the opposite handrim.

How a spotter can help

- Attach a spotter strap to the wheelchair as outlined in Section 1.9 Wheelies and stand behind the wheelchair user.
- Prevent the wheelchair from tipping backward.

Facing backward

With your wheelchair and a handrail

Only attempt this technique if you are very strong and have exceptionally good balance and wheelie skills.

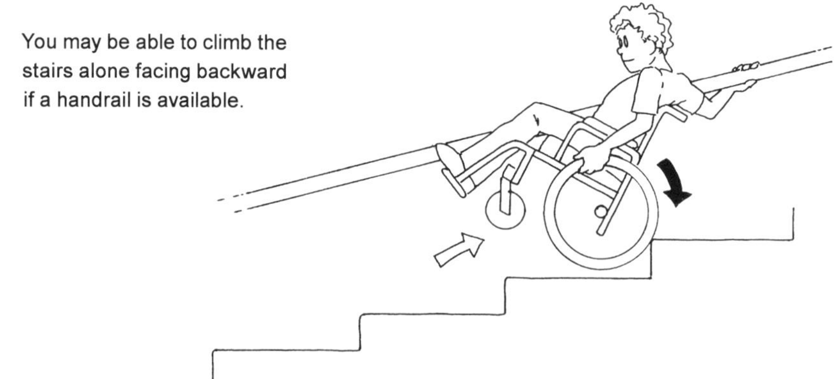

You may be able to climb the stairs alone facing backward if a handrail is available.

- It should be noted that this technique places the shoulder, of the arm reaching back to pull, in a biomechanically compromised position.
- Check the handrail for stability before using it. Handrails have been pulled off the wall using this technique.
- Back up to the stairs near one of the handrails until your rear wheels rest against the first step.
- Reach back and grab the handrail with the closest hand.
- With your free hand, pull back on the other handrim or reach across your body and grab the handrim nearest the handrail.
- Using the handrail as an anchor, tip yourself into a wheelie.
- Maintaining the wheelie position, pull on the handrail with one hand and pull backward on the handrim with the other hand. If you have the strength, this will move your wheelchair up one step at a time.
- Hold the tire steady as you slide your hand farther up the handrail.
- Pull on the handrail and push backward on the tire and/or handrim nearest the handrail again.
- Continue this motion until you reach the top of the stairs.
- Do not come out of the wheelie until you are far enough back from the top for the casters to come down on level ground and not off the edge of a step.

How a spotter can help

- Walk beside the wheelchair user.
- Prevent the wheelchair user from falling forward as well as tipping backward.

Without your wheelchair

If you cannot climb stairs in your wheelchair, you may be able to climb them without your wheelchair. This technique requires a significant amount of strength and balance. Wear a protective cushion inside your pants or strap one to your bottom to protect your skin when performing this technique. Do not scrape or rub against the steps as you go up.

- Maneuver close to the bottom step and transfer to the ground or one of the lower steps.
- Turn so your back is to the stairs.
- Place your hands up on the stair behind you.
- Raise your buttocks to the stair above by pushing up and back with your arms. Bending your head down can help lift your buttocks up as you lift to the next step.
- Bend your legs and position them on the stair below the one on which you are sitting.
- Repeat each step to move up the steps, repositioning your hands each time.
- Ask a helper to bring your wheelchair up for you.

You can bump yourself up a flight of stairs one step at a time. Wear a pressure relief cushion if you have no sensation in your sitting area.

Going Down Stairs with Assistance

You can go down stairs facing forward or backward. Unless the steps are long enough for the entire wheelchair to sit on all four wheels on the step you should strongly consider going down the steps backwards. At a minimum, the steps must be long enough to balance in a wheelie on each step. Decide which direction you want to face based on the number of steps, their slope, and the size of each landing.

With one assistant and a handrail going backward

- Check the handrail for stability. Handrails have been pulled off the wall using this technique.
- Position yourself so your back is to the stairs and your rear wheels are at the edge of the top step.
- Have your assistant stand a couple of steps below you with hands on the push handles or back support posts with the pull straps of your wheelchair.
- Grab the handrail with the nearest hand and hold a handrim with the other hand. Lean forward to maintain your balance.
- On your count of three, move your grip farther down the handrail while applying pressure to the handrim to slow yourself. At the same time, your assistant should lean into the back of your wheelchair while taking a step backward to lower you and your wheelchair slowly down one step. The assistant should not lean so hard that you are pushed back up the step.
- Another technique is to attach a climbing sling or a piece of rope or webbing near the top of the front caster around the frame of your wheelchair on each side of the chair.
- The front assistant puts tension up and forward on each of these straps as you count before rolling down to the next step. You should insist that your wheelchair roll down ONLY one step at a time. The assistant needs to step down to the next step while your wheelchair rests on that particular set of steps. This allows for you to re-grip the stairway handrail and your wheelchair handrim for the next count of three.
- Continue the process, step by step, until you reach the bottom of the stairs. As the front of your wheelchair slides down each step, the footrests may make a lot of noise.

With one assistant, no handrail and going backward

Only attempt this technique if your assistant is very strong and agile, and there is no handrail.

- Position yourself so your back is to the stairs and your rear wheels are at the edge of the top step.
- Have your assistant stand a couple of steps below you with hands on the push handles or back support posts with the pull straps.
- Lean forward and grasp both handrims.
- On your count of three, your assistant should take a step backward while leaning into the back of your wheelchair with just enough force to control your rate of descent. At the same time, you should help slow the descent by applying pressure to the handrims.
- Another technique is to attach a climbing sling or a piece of rope or webbing near the top of the front caster around the frame of your wheelchair on each side of the chair.
- The front assistant puts tension up and forward on each of these straps as you count before rolling down to the next

step. You should insist that your wheelchair roll down ONLY one step at a time. The assistant needs to step down to the next step while your wheelchair rests on that particular set of steps. This allows for you to re-grip your wheelchair handrim in preparation for the next count of three.

- As the front of your wheelchair slides down each step, your footrests may make a lot of noise.
- Continue the process until you reach the bottom of the stairs.

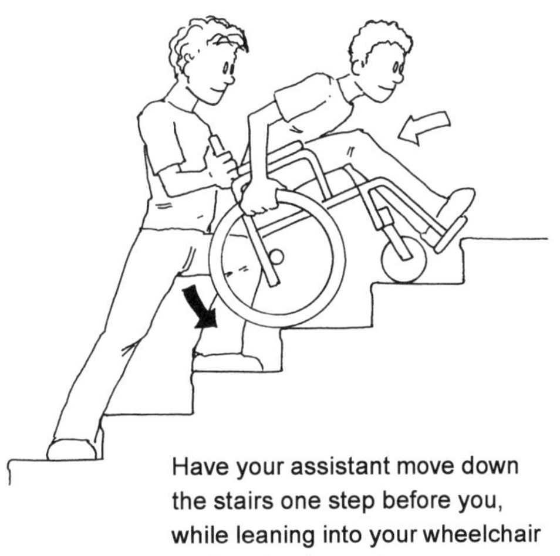

Have your assistant move down the stairs one step before you, while leaning into your wheelchair to slow the descent.

Going Down Stairs Alone

Descend stairs alone only if there are no assistants available. If the landing of each step is not long enough to accommodate your wheelchair's wheels, the stairs are too dangerous for you to ascend alone in your wheelchair. Regardless of how many times you have done this, it is a good idea to have a spotter in case you have a problem.

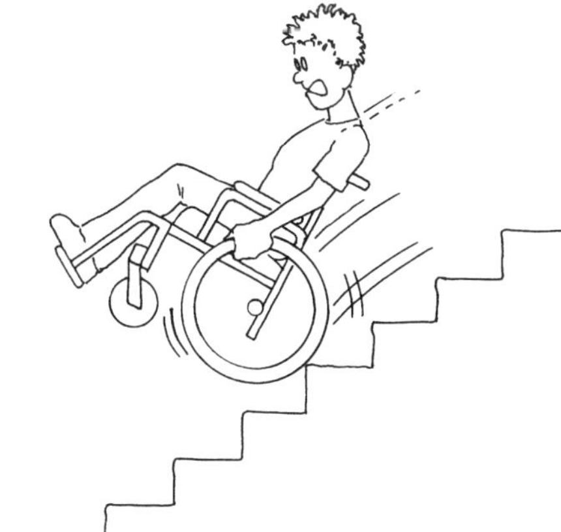

These stairs are too steep and short to descend alone safely.

Facing forward

Highest level of difficulty with the greatest level of balance and skill required

If the steps are few in number and deep enough to accommodate your rear wheels, you can descend them facing forward. Only attempt this technique if you are very skilled at balancing and moving in a wheelie.

- Make sure the steps are deep enough for your rear wheels to land and roll forward a bit.
- Face the stairs squarely so your wheels land on each step at the same time.
- Approach the stairs in a wheelie with your weight shifted back. You will be less likely to hurt yourself falling backward than tumbling forward down the stairs, so make sure to bring your weight back.
- Moving forward slowly, allow your rear wheels to roll onto the next step below.
- Drag on the handrims to slow your progress. You may want to come to a halt on each step to give yourself time to readjust.

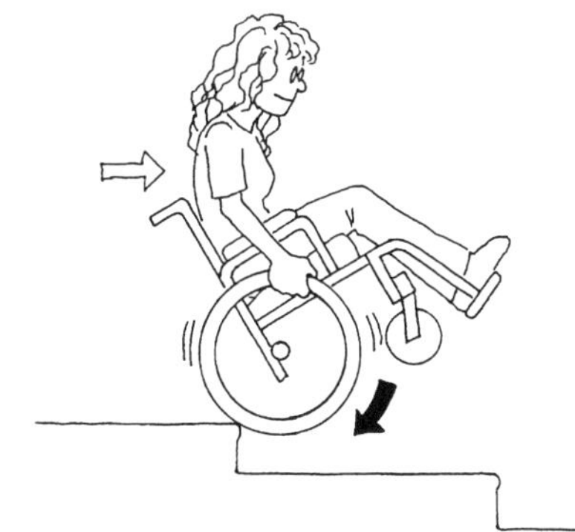

If the steps are deep enough and you have exceptional wheelie skills and balance, you can descend steps facing forward in a wheelie.

- Keep your hands on the wheels. If you reach for the handrail, your wheelchair will likely roll out from under you.

How a spotter can help

- Stand beside the wheelchair user.
- Spot the wheelchair user and prevent them from falling if the rider starts to fall forward or backward.

Descending backward

You may be able to manage steeper steps going backward. Only attempt this technique if you have a lap belt to secure yourself into the seat of your wheelchair.

Using one handrail

- Check the handrail for stability before using it. Handrails have been pulled off the wall using this technique.
- Lean forward, resting your chest on your knees.
- Be sure your wheelchair is square with the stairs. This will ensure that both wheels hit each step at the same time.
- Back your wheelchair toward the stairs, positioning your rear wheels as close to the edge as possible.
- Grab the handrail with the closest hand. Keep your other hand on the handrim.
- Lean forward, using the hand on the handrim to roll your wheelchair over the top step. Drag on the handrim will help slow you down. Do not get pulled out of your wheelchair.
- Hold onto the handrail, moving your hand down after you land on the step below.
- Continue with each step in this manner.

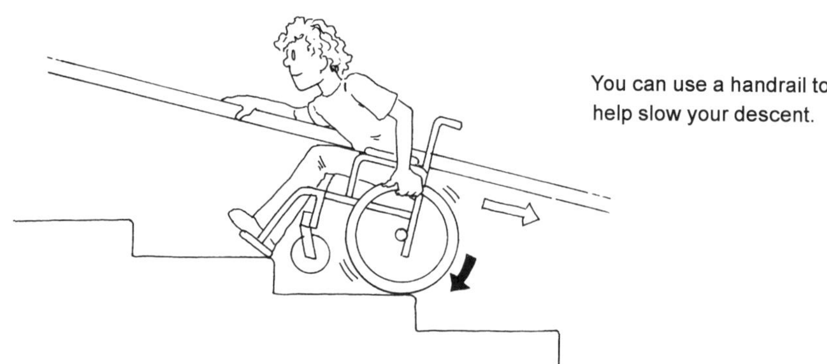

You can use a handrail to help slow your descent.

Using two handrails

- Only attempt this technique if you have a lap belt to secure yourself into the seat of your wheelchair.
- Check the handrails for stability before using them. Handrails have been pulled off the wall using this technique.
- Be sure your wheelchair is square with the stairs. This will ensure that both wheels hit each step at the same time.
- Back your wheelchair to the edge of the stairs.
- Grab onto the handrails.
- Lean forward, resting your chest on your knees.
- Allow your wheelchair to roll slowly backwards while you grip the handrails.
- Move your hands down after you land on the next step below.
- As the front of your wheelchair slides down each step, the footrests might make a lot of noise.
- Continue down each step in this manner.

Section 2.10

Elevators And Platform Lifts

The Americans with Disabilities Act (ADA) imposes strict guidelines that specify how elevators should be constructed to provide access to people with disabilities. These guidelines state that elevator doors should have a minimum width of 36 inches and remain open for at least five seconds. If the elevator doors close too quickly, ask the building manager to adjust the timing. (See Appendix A for information about the ADA.)

Catching an Elevator

Elevator banks

An "elevator bank," commonly found in places such as hotels and large office buildings, is a row of several elevators. When a person presses the call button, the next available elevator responds. Though this arrangement sounds convenient, you may find that if the elevator farthest from you opens, you might not be able to get to it before the doors close. To avoid this problem:

- Position yourself in the center of the elevator bank so you are close to all the elevators.
- Watch the floor indicators near or above each elevator. When the indicator number nears the floor you are on, prepare to catch that elevator.
- Keep pressing the call button until a closer elevator arrives.
- Ask someone to hold the elevator for you.

If all the elevators going your direction are full, you could take one going in the other direction and ride it until it changes directions. This often happens if you are on a lower floor such as two or three and want to go to the first floor. If the building has many floors, it could be full by the time it reaches you. You can wait for another elevator, but if they are continuously full, you may want to do something else. Take one going up, and you will be the first one on the elevator as it fills up going back down.

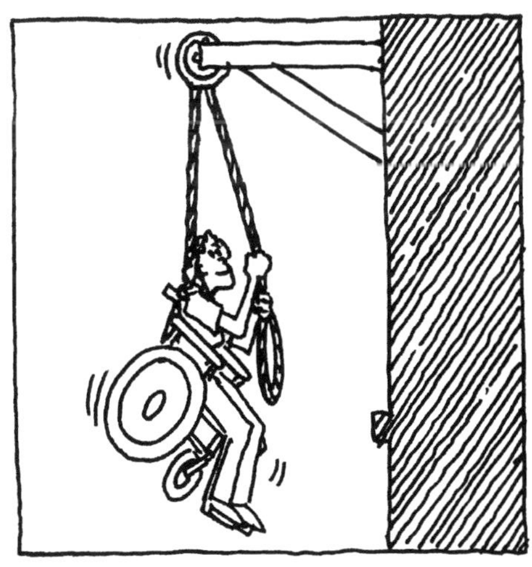

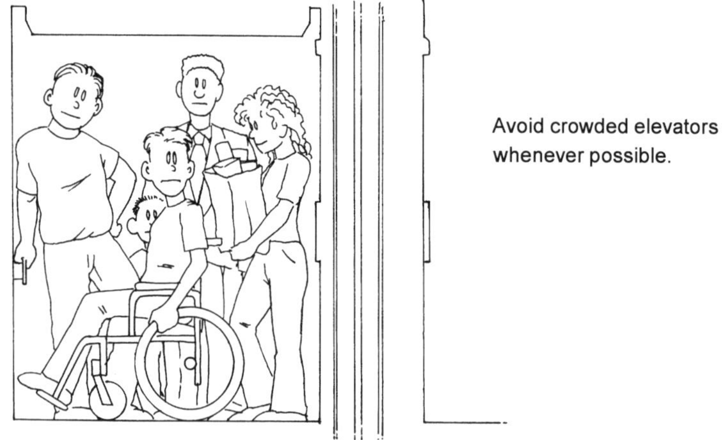

Avoid crowded elevators whenever possible.

Riding in an Elevator

Reaching elevator buttons

Sometimes the floor buttons inside the elevator and the call buttons outside of it are out of your reach. They may be too high or could be blocked by a plant, trash can or other object. Use a long object, such as a pen, pencil, reacher, flashlight, or other handy object, to push the button. If you do not have anything to push with, ask someone for help or try to move the object out of the way using your wheelchair as a plow. Mention the access problem to the building's management and suggest they move the obstacles. In some elevators, you might have to push the buttons when you're only partway through the door.

Some elevator cars are large and others are very small. If there is not enough room inside the elevator car to turn around, consider entering the elevator backwards. By entering backwards, it will likely be easier for you to reach the call buttons inside the elevator and it will be easier for you to move into position to exit the elevator when it reaches your floor.

Negotiating elevator-to-floor gaps

Elevators are supposed to stop within a half inch of the floor, but if there is a wide vertical or horizontal gap between the elevator car and the building's floor, negotiate gaps of less than two inches as you would a threshold or curb. (See Sections 2.2 and 2.8 for more information about thresholds and curbs.) If the gap is larger than two inches, wait for another elevator rather than risk a hazardous entry.

The following section describes how to enter an elevator car that is either above (approaching a rise) or below (approaching a drop) the level of the floor. The maneuvers are the same as ascending or descending small curbs. If you are just learning, you can practice on a small curb so you don't have to deal with the timing of the closing elevator door.

Approach a rise facing forward

- Shift your weight back and propel your caster wheels onto the rise or pop your caster up slightly to climb the small obstacle.
- Without losing momentum, keep moving forward until your rear wheels move up onto the rise and you are fully in the elevator.

Approaching a rise facing backward

- Watch for people or obstacles that may be behind you.
- Propel your rear wheels up onto the rise.
- Without losing momentum, keep moving backward until your caster wheels move onto the rise and your wheelchair has moved fully into the elevator.

Approaching a drop facing forward

- Shift your weight back and propel forward until your front wheels drop to the lower surface. Be careful that you don't tip or fall forward as your front caster wheels drop to the lower surface.

- Without losing momentum, continue moving forward until your rear wheels drop to the lower surface and your wheelchair rolls fully into the elevator.

Approaching a drop facing backward

- Lean forward and slowly propel backward until your rear wheels land on the lower surface.
- Continue moving backward until your front wheels drop to the lower surface and your wheelchair moves fully into the elevator.

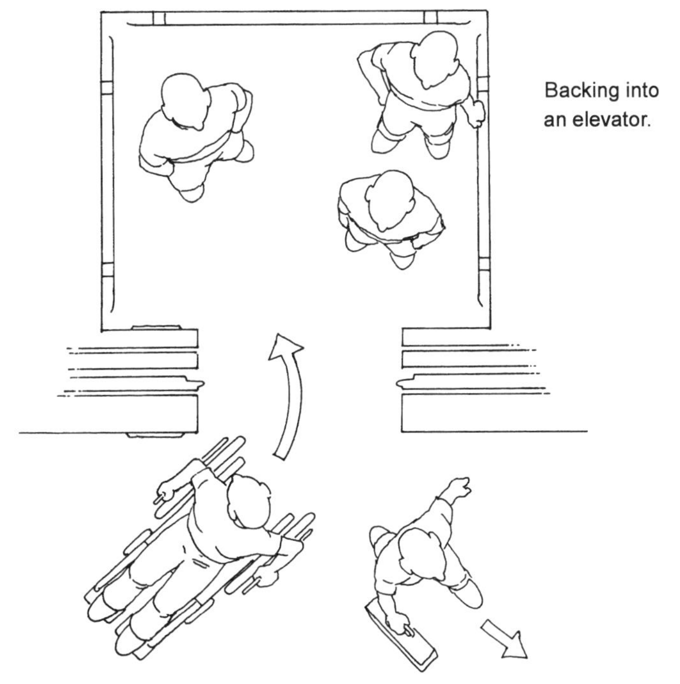

Backing into an elevator.

Positioning Yourself in an Elevator

Uncrowded elevators

Facing forward

- Enter the elevator facing forward, looking for rises or drops as you cross from the floor to the elevator.
- Turn around inside the elevator to face the door.
- Exit the elevator facing forward, staying alert for other people, rises or drops to floor level, or other obstacles.

Entering backward

If you are riding the elevator with someone, ask him or her to hold the door so you can back into the elevator from outside. There is more room to maneuver outside the elevator than inside. If you back into the elevator, make sure you know if there is a rise or drop to get in.

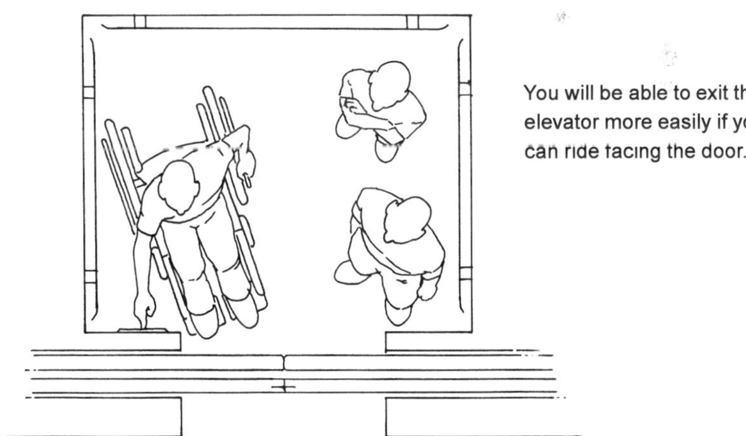

You will be able to exit the elevator more easily if you can ride facing the door.

Crowded elevators

It is usually easier to enter a crowded elevator facing forward. You will be able to see where you are going and others can avoid your foot supports and hang over the front of your chair. Backing in can be difficult for people to get out of the way of your tires.

- Enter the elevator facing forward, watching for rises or drops to the elevator floor.
- Stay in this position until you reach your floor.
- Exit the elevator facing backward. Be sure to look behind you for other people, rises or drops to floor level, and obstacles.

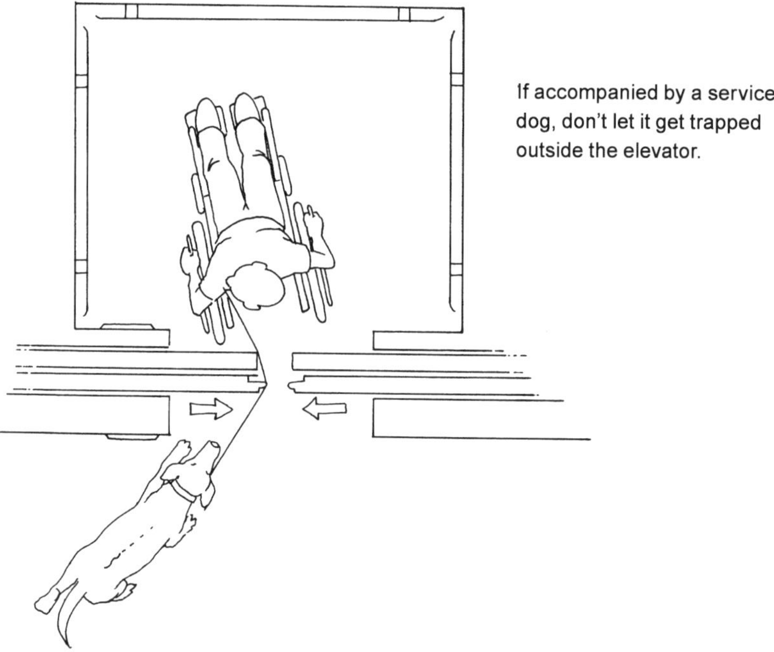

If accompanied by a service dog, don't let it get trapped outside the elevator.

Out of service elevators

Find or call the front desk or main office. They may be able to repair the elevator or direct you to an alternative elevator, such as a freight elevator or one specified for employees.

If you are on a high floor in a building, there may be an attendant driven evacuation track system that will carry you and your wheelchair down the stairway. If you regularly use an elevator and your office is upstairs, you might want to find out if the building has evacuation chairs that are designed to take you down the stairway with assistance in the event of an emergency when the elevators are not working. Safety and performance standards now exist for the safety and performance of evacuation chairs and are available from RESNA.org.

If you are riding mass transportation and the only elevator at the transit stop is out of service, you are usually entitled to ride to another station and to take a taxi to your destination at the transit company's expense.

Emergency communication systems

Most elevators have an emergency communication system. Use this phone or other device to summon help in an emergency. Be familiar with the emergency communication system in elevators you use on a regular basis.

If you find a problem with the system, notify the management immediately to initiate repairs. Some common problems:

- The door to the box is difficult to open
- The communication device is missing or out of order
- The cord is too short (it should be at least 29 inches long)
- The unit is out of your reach
- It also helps to carry a cell phone if you need assistance.

Platform Lifts

Some buildings have platform lifts instead of ramps or elevators to carry wheelchair users to another level. The metal platform functions like a van lift. These lifts should not be locked but are sometimes locked and you will have to find the person with the key and notify the building manager that they need to make provisions for the lift to work without the requirement for a key.

Riding on platform lifts

When learning to ride on platform lifts, practice with a spotter nearby. Ask him or her to make sure all four of your tires are safely on the platform before you move the lift.

Most platform lifts are constructed so you can roll forward to enter and can continue rolling forward to exit. If the lift requires you to use the same door to enter and leave, consider backing onto the lift. This way, you can roll forward when exiting.

- Roll onto the lift, making sure all four of your tires are safely on the platform.
- Set your wheel locks.
- Press the button to raise or lower the lift.
- Wait until the lift has come to a complete stop at the top or bottom before releasing your wheel locks.
- Exit the lift.

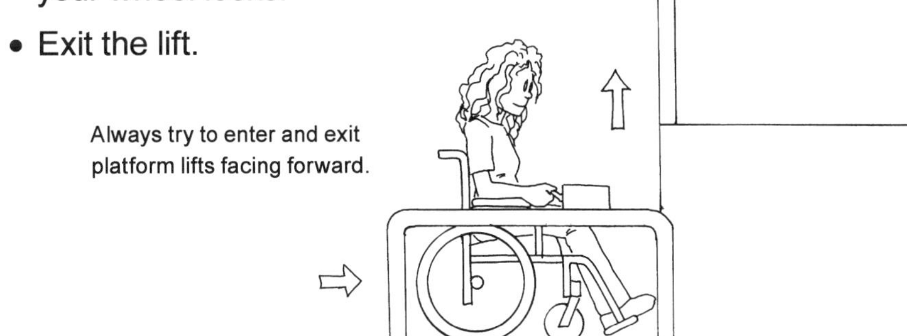

Always try to enter and exit platform lifts facing forward.

How to ask for assistance

- If you are unsure about how to operate the lift, ask someone to help you.
- Ask an assistant to make sure all four of your tires are safely on the platform.
- An assistant can help with the doors on the lift by meeting you at the top or bottom.

How a spotter can help

- Stand in a position that enables you to make sure all four of the wheelchair tires are safely on the lift and also make sure the wheelchair user doesn't lose their balance if the platform tilts as it rises or lowers.

Section 2.11

Escalators

Most buildings that contain escalators also have elevators. Always opt to use an elevator before an escalator because escalators pose many hazards to wheelchair users. Only use an escalator if you have no other means of reaching a particular destination. Some public accommodations do not permit wheelchairs on escalators. These entities have a right to deny you access to the escalator if an elevator or ramp is available.

Only perform the techniques in this section if you absolutely must use an escalator in an emergency and there is no other accessible alternative available. These techniques require a significant amount of wheelchair experience and strength to accomplish, and may expose you and any assistants to physical strain and serious injury. Read the warning on page vi to learn about the risks involved in performing wheelchair skills. Falling on an escalator is especially dangerous and may result in severe injury or death!

Before practicing the techniques in this chapter, you should be able to shift your weight forward, propel your wheelchair forward and backward, and have enough strength and dexterity to grip escalator rails securely. Always practice and perform escalator skills with an assistant.

Always observe an escalator before riding it to see whether the steps can safely accommodate your wheels. If the escalator handrails have patterns or other identifiable marks in them, try to determine whether the rails move at the same rate as the steps. Do not ride escalators that do not run smoothly or have jerky handrails.

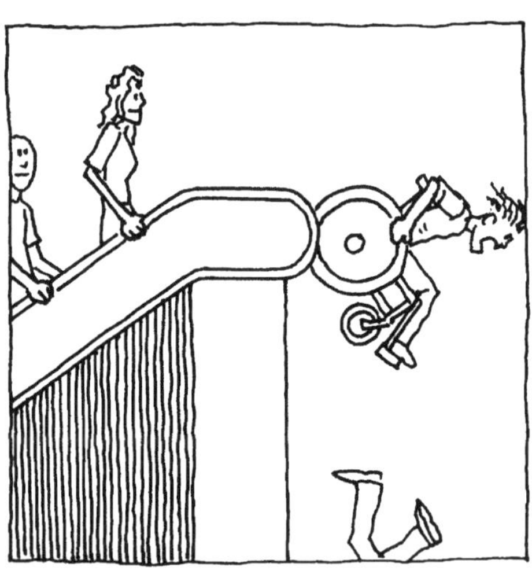

Going Up an Escalator with Assistance

- Roll forward onto the escalator platform.
- Position yourself so that when the steps begin to appear, your rear wheels are on the flat portion rather than the edge of a step. Watch the steps as they rise up and roll yourself forward or backward as needed. Roll your rear wheels to sit out toward the edge of a step, while rolling firmly forward against the face of a rising step.

- Your foot support will be positioned on one step and your rear wheels down two steps with an empty escalator step between them. Depending on the escalator and your wheelchair setup, your front caster wheels will either rest on or dangle above the middle step.
- Use one hand to grip a handrail and the other to grip your wheelchair handrim.
- Lean forward to avoid tipping over backward.
- If the escalator steps are too shallow to accommodate your rear wheels, brace them against the vertical surface of the step above.
- Grab onto the escalator handrails. They will pull you forward and onto the escalator. Be careful they don't pull you out of your wheelchair.
- If the handrails move faster than the steps, let the rail slide through your hand so your arm stays with your wheelchair. If the handrails move slower than the steps, apply pressure to your handrim to avoid slipping backward as you move your other hand forward on the moving handrail to keep up with your wheels.
- Have an assistant follow you onto the escalator with one foot one step below you and bracing with the other foot two steps below you. Your assistant should be facing upward with hands resting lightly on the push handles or back support posts with the pull straps of your wheelchair to prevent you from rolling backward. Your assistant should not put pressure on your wheelchair unless you begin to tip or slide backward down the escalator.
- As the escalator steps level out at the top, gradually sit upright to maintain your balance. Once all four of your wheels are at the same level and the stairs have leveled out you will need to propel your wheelchair forward. Most wheelchair riders prefer to keep their dominant hand pulling against the moving handrail and keep their other hand on the wheelchair handrim to push forward off of the steps as they become flush. Keep in mind that you have to roll from a moving conveyor up onto a stationary transition plate, which is the equivalent of rolling forward across a low profile door threshold. Once clear of the moving handrail, use your wheelchair handrims to keep your wheelchair moving forward away from the escalator.
- Your assistant's hands should remain near the push handles or back support posts with the pull straps until you are safely off and clear of the escalator.

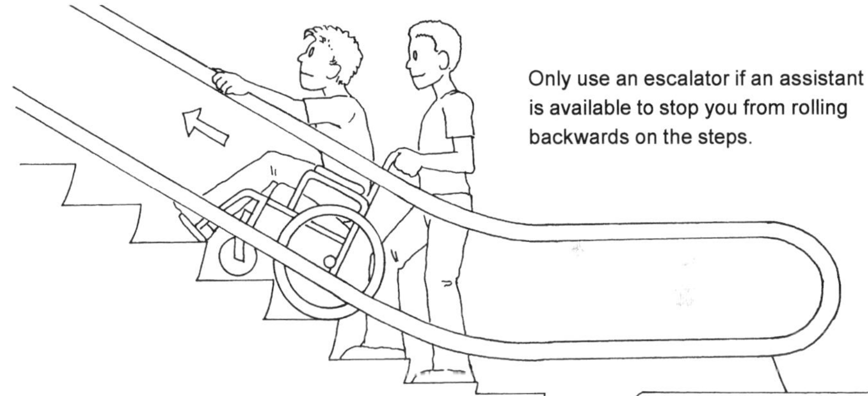

Only use an escalator if an assistant is available to stop you from rolling backwards on the steps.

Going Down an Escalator with Assistance

- Ask your assistant to step onto the escalator before you and stand facing upward. When you roll backward onto the escalator, your assistant should stand one step below your rear wheels and prevent you from rolling or tipping backward.

- Roll backward onto the escalator until your rear wheels are one step lower than your front caster wheels. Watch the steps as they rise up and roll forward or backward as needed so that you can roll your rear wheels to sit out toward the edge of a step but can roll firmly forward against the face of a rising step.
- Lean forward and grasp one handrail as high as possible. Apply pressure to your wheelchair handrim with the other hand to avoid slipping backward.
- Your assistant's hands should be on your wheelchair's push handles or back support posts with the pull straps.
- Push your wheelchair forward so the rear wheels are secure on a step.
- Your assistant should make sure you do not roll or tip over backward.
- When you reach the bottom, wait for the steps to level out. Most wheelchair riders prefer to push back on the moving handrail with their dominant hand and keep their other hand on the wheelchair handrim to roll back off the steps as they become flush. Keep in mind that you have to roll from a moving conveyor up onto a stationary transition plate, which is the equivalent of rolling backwards across a low profile door threshold. Once clear of the moving handrail, use your wheelchair handrims to roll back and away from the escalator.
- Your assistant's hands should remain on the push handles or back support posts with the pull straps until you reach the bottom of the escalator and all four of your wheels are off of and clear of the escalator. Be sure your assistant backs up as you reach the escalator platform so you can reverse off the escalator.

Section 2.12

Tracks and Grates

Always examine railroad tracks and grates before you cross them. On railroad tracks, determine how far the rails protrude above the sidewalk surface and estimate the width of the spaces between the rails and the sidewalk surface. On grates, determine if the drainage slots are wider than your wheels. Your caster wheels could easily get stuck in these gaps, so try to cross in a wheelie or at the very least, perpendicular to railroad tracks or grates. If you cross on four wheels and your caster wheels swivel sideways, they could get stuck in the gaps. Also, determine if your anti-tip device or foot support clearance will be a problem.

Have a spotter nearby to help you when crossing railroad and trolley tracks so you will not get stuck halfway across. Having a spotter is especially important when crossing tracks unfamiliar to you. If a spotter is helping you negotiate tracks or grates, use a spotter strap as described and explained in Section 1.9 Wheelies.

Before practicing the techniques in this section, you should be able to propel a wheelchair forward and backward and be able to cross obstacles. You will be able to cross railroad tracks and grates more easily if you can pop a wheelie and move forward in a wheelie position.

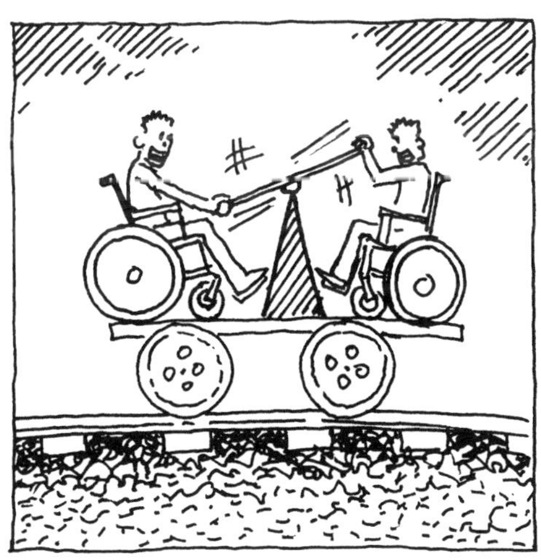

Crossing Railroad and Trolley Tracks

Look at the track and determine if you can cross safely. Unless someone is available to help you if you get stuck, do not cross the track if you have any doubts about your safety.

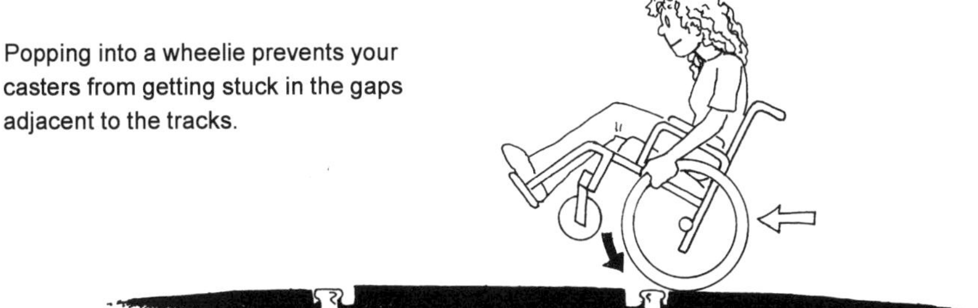

Popping into a wheelie prevents your casters from getting stuck in the gaps adjacent to the tracks.

In a wheelie

- As you approach the railroad tracks, pop a wheelie.
- Maintaining the wheelie position, move forward across the railroad tracks.
- Try to cross perpendicular to the railroad tracks so your rear tires cross at the same time.
- Wait until you have cleared the railroad tracks before lowering yourself out of the wheelie position.

On four wheels

If you are unable to pop a wheelie, try crossing railroad tracks on four wheels. Do not deviate from a path perpendicular to the railroad tracks because any turning motion could cause your caster wheels to fall into the gaps on either side of the tracks and get stuck. Section 1.5 has more information about caster wheel management.

- Look at the railroad track and determine if you can cross safely. Unless someone is available to help you if you get stuck, do not cross the track if you have any doubts about your safety.
- Slowly propel forward across the railroad tracks. Position your wheelchair so you cross perpendicular to the tracks, without changing direction. This will reduce the risk of the caster wheels dropping into the gaps adjacent to the tracks.
- There are often dips in the asphalt on either side of railroad tracks which can also be hazardous. Move slowly to avoid getting stuck, losing your balance or tipping.

If your caster turns sideways, it could get caught in a crevice and stop your wheelchair.

How a spotter can help

- Attach a spotter strap to the wheelchair or walk behind the wheelchair user with hands close to the push handles to prevent the wheelchair user from tipping over.

How to ask for assistance

- Because anti-tip devices and foot supports can also catch on tracks and get stuck in the surrounding channels, you may want to ask an assistant to adjust them to their non-effective position before crossing a set of tracks.
- It may be easiest for an assistant to pull you across tracks backward in a wheelie to prevent the foot supports from getting caught and tipping you out of your wheelchair.
- Turn so your back is to the tracks.
- Ask your assistant to stand behind your wheelchair and hold the push handles or back support posts with the pull straps. Together with your assistant, tip your wheelchair back into a wheelie position by having your assistant stand sideways to push a hip into the back of your wheelchair.

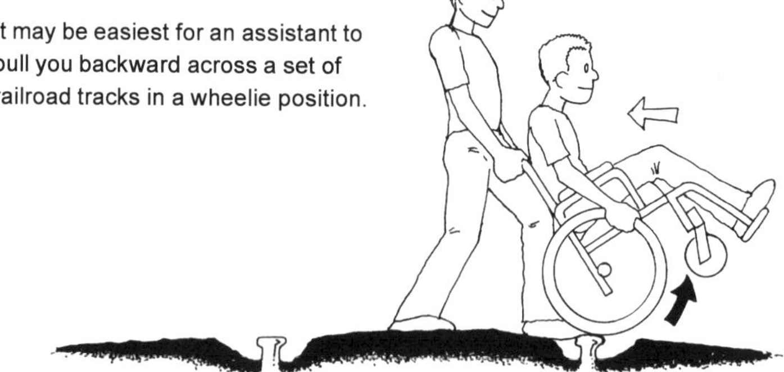

It may be easiest for an assistant to pull you backward across a set of railroad tracks in a wheelie position.

- On your count of three, pull on your handrims and/or tires while your assistant pulls back on the push handles. Be sure your assistant uses leg rather than back strength.
- Only come out of the wheelie position after you have crossed the railroad tracks.

Helpful Hint

Secure any loose belongings before crossing grates or railroad tracks. The uneven surfaces around grates and tracks could jostle your keys or other belongings out of a pocket and onto the ground.

Crossing Grates

Whether you live in the city or the country, you are likely to encounter sewer or cattle grates. Grates should be positioned so the longer openings are perpendicular to the most common path of travel. Grate openings should not be more than half an inch wide in one direction. Since many grates do not meet these standards, it's best to avoid crossing directly over them whenever possible. If you must cross a grate, go slowly and plot a course perpendicular to the grate slots.

With a spotter, practice crossing different grates. You can often find grates on city sidewalks and at the base of driveways and ramps.

Wide slots and a lack of crossbars make cattle guards extreme versions of sewer grates. As with all grates, cross a cattle guard perpendicular to the bars. Exceptional balance and control in a wheelie are required to cross cattle guards.

The easiest way to cross a grate is to pop a wheelie to prevent your caster wheels from getting caught in the grate slots. As with railroad tracks, the openings in grates can easily catch your caster wheels. Crossing grates in a wheelie will also make the crossing smoother.

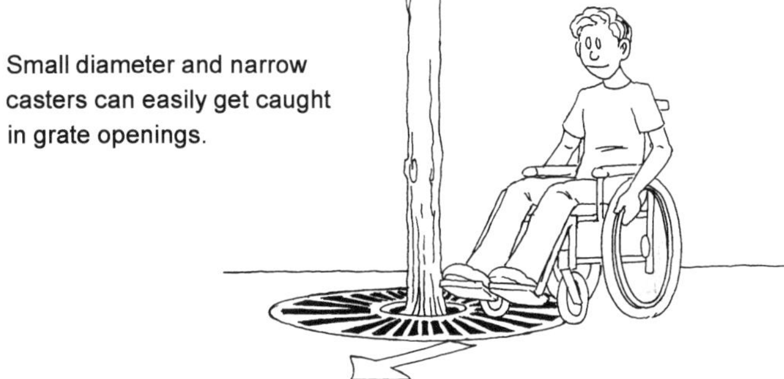

Slots perpendicular to or narrower than your rear tires

- As you approach the grate, pop a wheelie.
- In the wheelie, move forward over the grate.
- Remain in the wheelie until you have cleared the grate.

Slots parallel to or wider than your rear tires

- As you approach the gate, pop a wheelie.
- In the wheelie, turn your chair perpendicular to the grate and cross it.
- Remain in the wheelie until you have cleared the grate.

How to ask for assistance

- Together with your assistant, tip your wheelchair back into the wheelie position. Ask your assistant to stand behind your wheelchair and hold onto the push handles or back support posts with the pull straps. Have your assistant turn sideways and push a hip into the back of your wheelchair, tipping you backward until you are in a wheelie position.
- When you are ready, ask your assistant to push. You may want to help by pushing forward on your handrims.
- When crossing large grates, like cattle guards or railroad crossings, always have your assistant roll you backwards across the obstruction.
- When you have cleared the grate, lean forward and ask your assistant to lower your wheelchair.
- Sometimes it is easier for your assistant to help you over a grate like this by rolling your wheelchair backward. Have the assistant pop your wheelchair into a wheelie before rolling you backwards over the grate.

How a spotter can help

- Walk behind the wheelchair user to prevent him or her from tipping backward or losing forward balance.

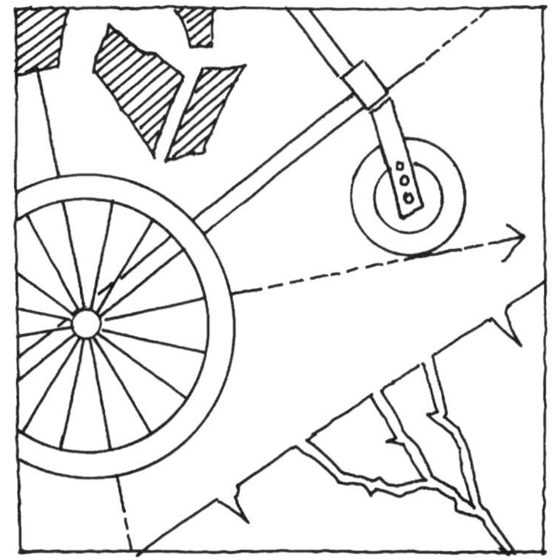

Chapter 3

Sections in This Chapter

Emergency Skills

Fire! The smoke is rising fast to your floor, and the incandescent glow of flames has reached the floor below you. People are screaming, choking in the smoke, and running down the fire escapes. You rush to the hall and the elevators are dead. What do you do now?

The stress and panic of an emergency can make it difficult to think clearly and act wisely. Practice disaster and safety procedures in advance so that you will be calmer and react appropriately in an actual emergency. If you are active in your wheelchair, chances are that you will need to use your emergency skills at some point.

Read the warning on page vi to learn about the risks involved in performing wheelchair skills. Falling is an unacceptable option for some wheelchair users that may result in severe injury or death.

Section 3.1

Falling and Getting Up

Learning how to fall without getting hurt and how to get back into your wheelchair are important safety skills. It is best to learn these skills with the coaching and supervision of a physical or occupational therapist who has wheelchair training experience in a rehabilitation environment. As a wheelchair user, you should know how to fall and get up, or be able to instruct others to help you get back into your wheelchair.

The skills in this section may expose you and any assistants helping you to physical strain and serious injury. Read the warning on page vi to learn about the risks involved in performing wheelchair skills. Falling is an unacceptable option for some wheelchair users that may result in severe injury or death.

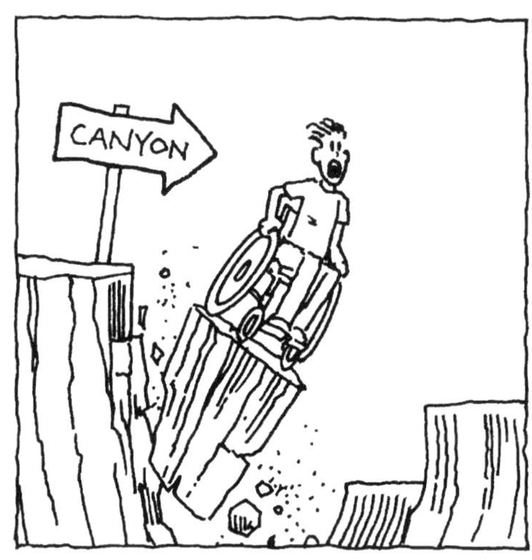

Falling

When learning to fall safely, always practice on a soft surface such as a mat, soft carpet, futon, or soft sand.

Practice fall

- Have a spotter stand behind your wheelchair with his or her hands on the push handles or back posts, or using a spotting strap.
- Tip your wheelchair into the wheelie position. If necessary, ask your spotter to help tip your wheelchair back into a wheelie.
- When you are ready, have the spotter lower you backward to the ground. Tuck your chin into your chest and hold your knees. Make sure the spotter bends his or her knees, maintains a straight back, and uses his or her legs for strength. (See Section 5.1 for more information about preventing back injuries.)

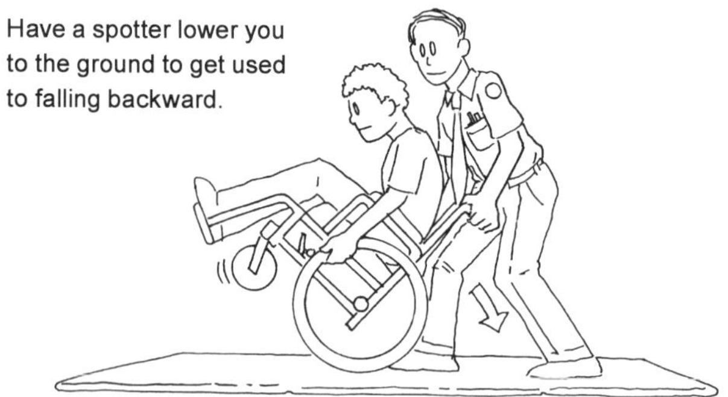
Have a spotter lower you to the ground to get used to falling backward.

Falling backward

- Always protect your head!
- If you start falling backward, tuck your chin into your chest. This will prevent your head from hitting the ground first.
- Hold your knees back with both hands or keep them away from your face with your arm.
- Try slowing the fall by reaching back to the floor with one hand.
- Accessories such as push handles and backpacks might help by preventing the back support of your wheelchair from hitting the ground.

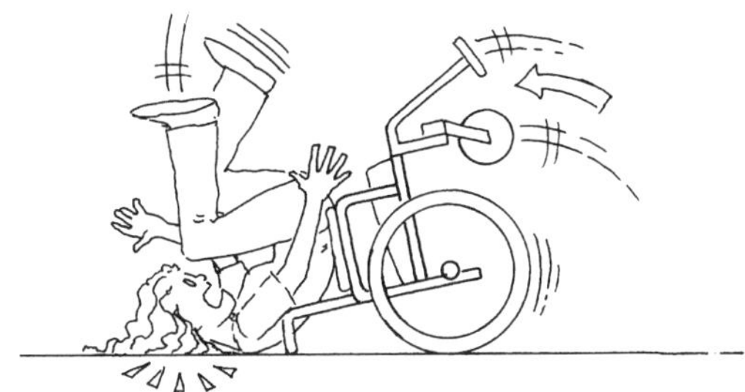

If you fall backward and don't take preventive actions, your head will hit the ground and your knees will fall back and hit your face.

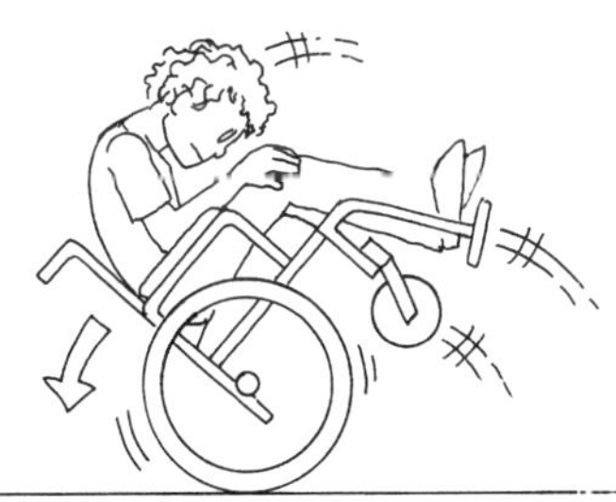

Tuck your chin to your chest and hold at least one arm over your legs. If you don't hold your legs they may fall back into your face and hurt you.

How a spotter can help

- Stand behind the wheelchair with your hands on the push handles,on the back support posts, or holding onto the pull straps.
- When the wheelchair user is ready, tip the chair into a wheelie.
- Then, turn your body sideways and push a hip into the back of the wheelchair.
- To avoid back injuries, don't twist at the waist.
- Lower the wheelchair to the floor.

Falling forward

- Ask someone you know that is comfortable performing a shoulder roll to demonstrate one for you. If you find yourself being thrown from your wheelchair to the right, try to pull your right arm across your body toward the opposite shoulder and turn and tuck your head downward toward the same opposite shoulder. You want to try and curl into a ball so you will roll out of your wheelchair instead of landing on the ground face first.
- Putting your arms out in front of you to stop your fall can result in a broken arm or wrist.

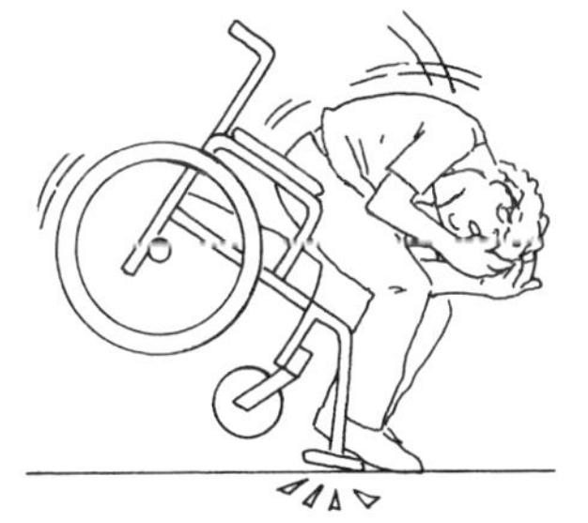

Curl into a ball and tuck your chin and shoulder to the side to roll out of your wheelchair during a forward fall.

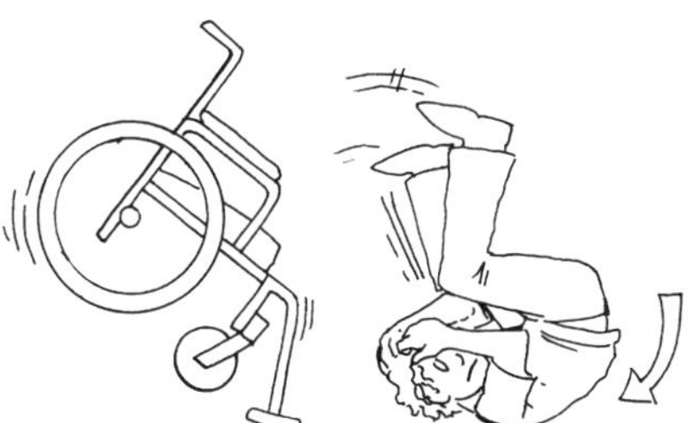

Falling sideways

- Lean in the opposite direction of the fall to prevent your head from hitting the ground.
- Place both arms on the arm support or wheel in the opposite direction of the fall so the chair hits the ground before you do. Do not catch yourself by reaching out an arm because you could injure your wrist, elbow, or shoulder. Reaching out could also cause the wheelchair to land on your arm or hand resulting in greater injury.
- If you do reach with your arm, keep it bent so it can serve as a shock absorber. Do not let this arm get caught underneath your wheelchair as you fall.

Getting Up

Before getting up

- Make sure you have not broken any bones or hurt yourself in any other way.
- Be sure all your "plumbing" (leg bag, catheter, etc.) is in place.
- Check for damage to your wheelchair. Make sure all parts are in their proper positions, including your arm supports, leg supports, back support, and any cushions you use before climbing back into your wheelchair.
- You may want to put your seat cushion on the ground and sit on it to reduce the distance you have to lift yourself back into your wheelchair.
- If you are on a slope, position your wheelchair sideways across the slope and lock your wheel locks if you can. This will help prevent your wheelchair from rolling downhill.
- Be sure the caster wheels are trailing forward to increase your wheelchair's forward stability. (See Section 1.5 for more information on caster trail.)

Getting up from a fall

There are different ways to get up from a fall. The technique you find easiest will depend on the situation, your level of injury, your strength, and the amount of assistance available.

When learning to get up from a fall, have a spotter stand behind your wheelchair to brace it. The spotter can retrieve a wheelchair escaping down a hill and help lift you if necessary.

Facing your wheelchair

- Be sure your caster wheels are trailing forward. You may want to remove your seat cushion from the wheelchair so the seat support surface of your wheelchair is lower.
- Lock your wheels. If you do not have wheel locks, try to brace the back of your wheelchair against a firm object such as a wall or couch to keep it from rolling away as you climb into it. If there is someone available to hold your wheelchair ask them to hold the push handles or back support tubes.
- Bend your knees to one side and face your wheelchair.
- Grasp the frame of the wheelchair in the front, where the caster wheels are attached.
- Pull yourself into a kneeling position and lean forward onto the seat of your wheelchair. Push up with your hands, pulling your legs forward, until your knees are on or near the foot supports.
- With another, stronger push, lift yourself up and hold on to the back of your wheelchair. It may help to hook your chin over the back support.

- Reach up with one arm to hold onto a push handle, back support, arm support or other stable part of the frame.
- Roll yourself to the side, until you drop into a seated position.
- Adjust yourself into a comfortable position. Do not forget to slip your seat cushion back underneath you. Be sure your feet are on the foot supports.

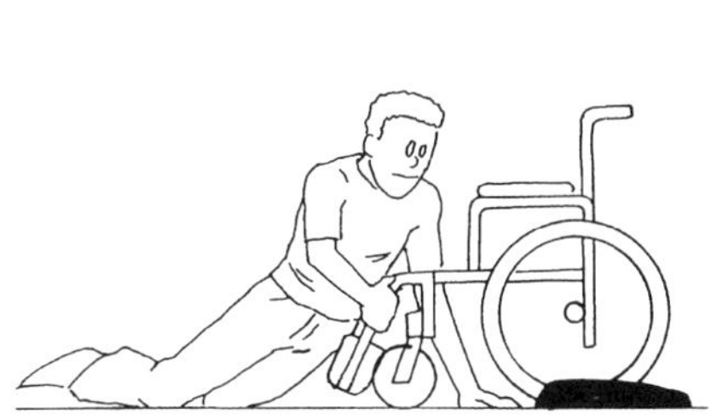

1. After righting your wheelchair, lay with your knees bent to the side in front of the footrests.

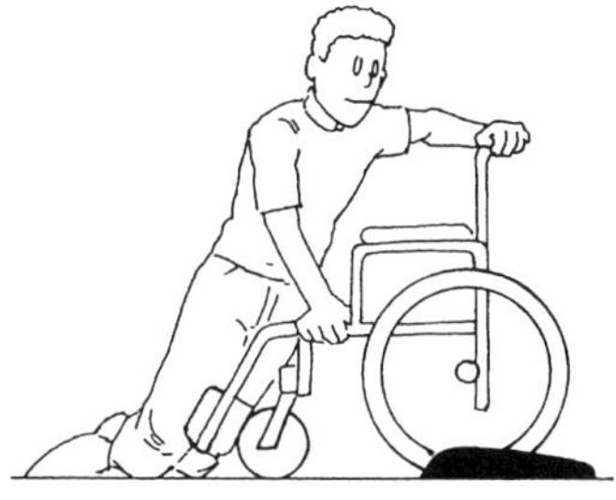

2. Rest your knees on or near the foot supports.

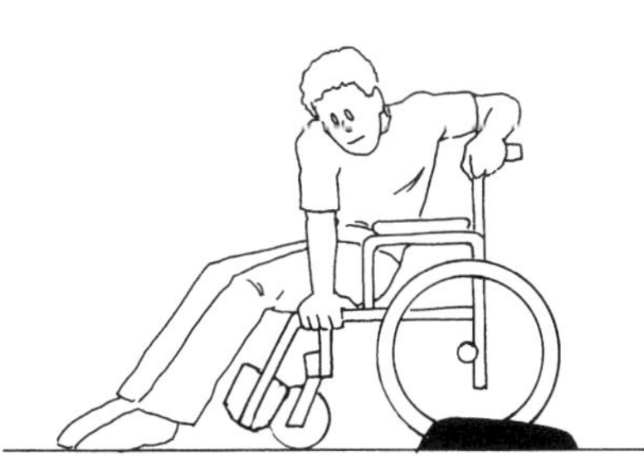

3. Pull yourself up and onto your wheelchair seat.

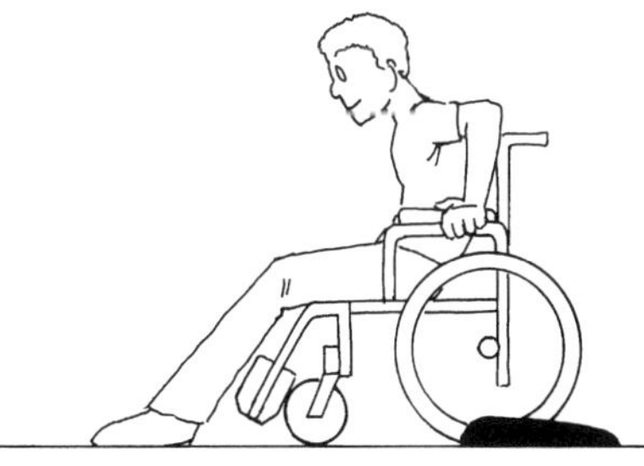

4. Twist yourself around until you are sitting upright.

Facing away from your wheelchair – Not Recommended

- This is an older technique that someone may try to teach you. It is not recommended.
- Note that this technique requires you to reach behind your body and extend your elbows up above the level of your shoulder.
- Any transfer that requires you to have your elbow above the height of your shoulder puts your shoulder into a compromising position. Your shoulder is only held together by the rotator cuff group of muscles. Using your shoulders to lift your body in this position may injure one or more of your rotator cuff muscles or tendons.

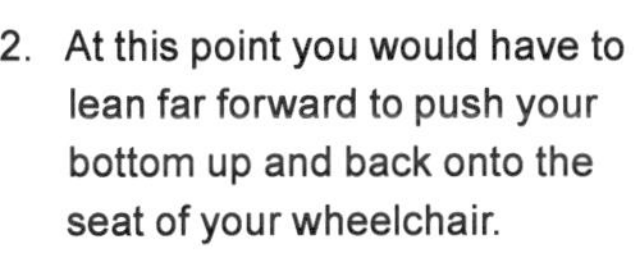

1. Reaching behind your body with your elbows above your shoulder during any transfer is a bad idea. This places your shoulder in a position that may result in injury to one or more of your rotator cuff muscles or tendons.

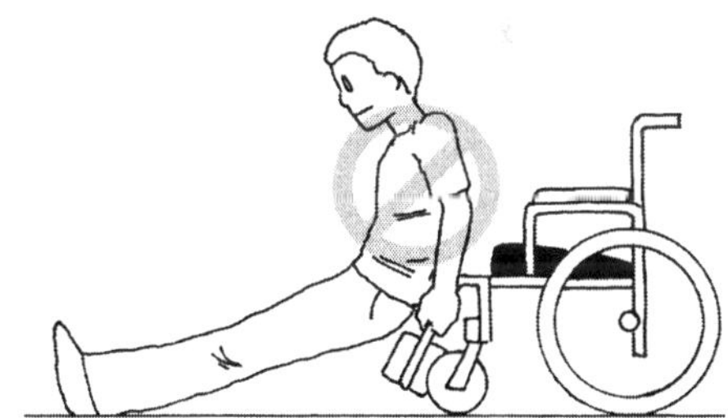

2. At this point you would have to lean far forward to push your bottom up and back onto the seat of your wheelchair.

Side-to-side technique

- Sit on your cushion at an angle to your wheelchair. This will elevate your body off of the floor, decreasing the height of the transfer up to the seat support surface of your wheelchair.

- Grab the frame on the far side of your wheelchair just in front of the seat support surface of your wheelchair.
- Position your bent knees between your wheelchair's frame and your outside arm.
- Lean your head and trunk forward on your knees, pushing down with the hand on your seat cushion and flex your elbow while pulling yourself forward with the hand that is holding onto the frame of your wheelchair.
- With the weight of your chest on your knees, tip forward as far as possible to get your bottom up in the air.
- Pivot your body and sit in your wheelchair seat.
- Slip your seat cushion back underneath you. Be sure your feet are on the foot supports.

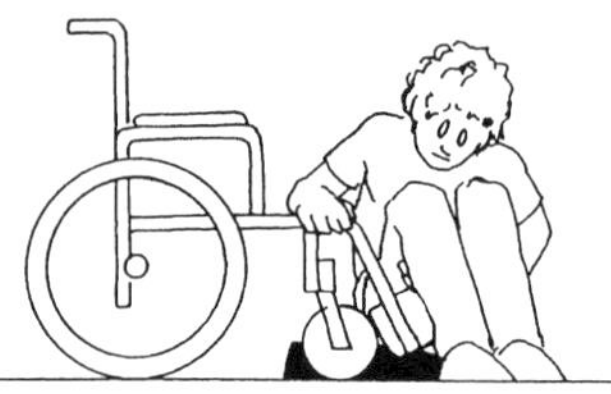

1. Grasp the frame of the wheelchair just in front of the seat support surface of your wheelchair while sitting on your cushion.

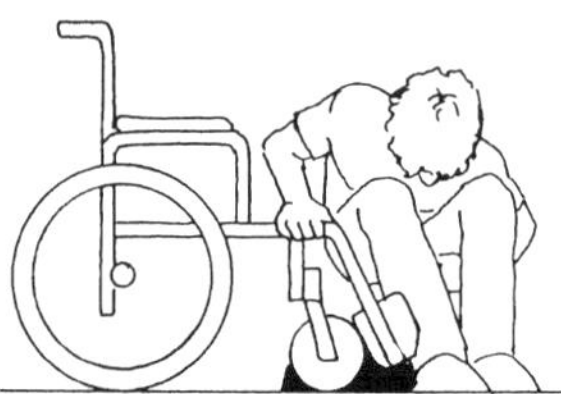

2. Push down on the hand on your seat cushion and flex your elbow while pulling yourself forward with the hand that is holding onto the frame of the wheelchair.

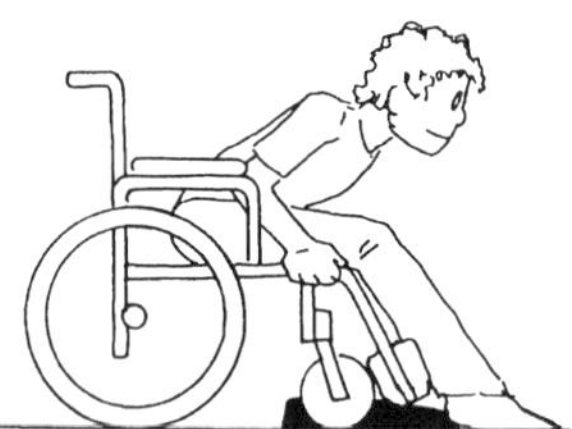

3. Lean forward with your weight on your chest and your head down and then pivot your body into the seat of your wheelchair.

How to ask for assistance

Using an assistant to help is sometimes the safest, quickest, easiest, and most convenient way to get back in your wheelchair. (Read Section 5.1 for more information about assisting safely.) There are several methods to help someone into a wheelchair.

With an assistant pushing up

- Rotate the caster wheels until they are trailing forward.
- Engage your wheel locks.
- With your back to your wheelchair, reach behind and put your hands on the frame where the foot supports are attached. Do not use this method if your elbows are above the height of your shoulders. Do not use this method if your shoulders do not feel strong while lifting in this position.
- Have your assistant place their hands securely under your knees.
- On your count of three, have your assistant lift you at the knees, while you push up and back until you are sitting in your wheelchair.

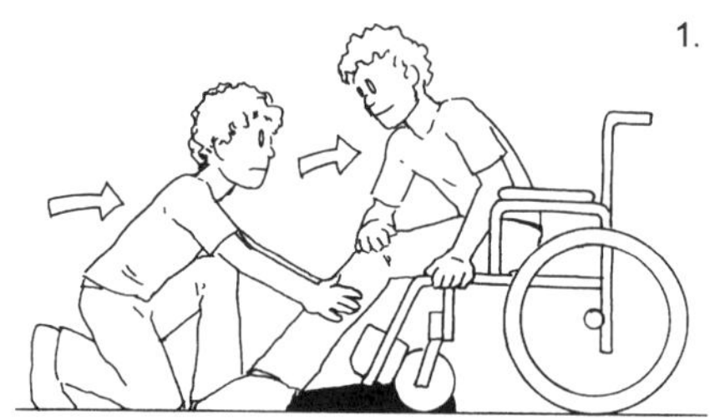

1. Have your assistant lift you by the knees as you push down with your arms.

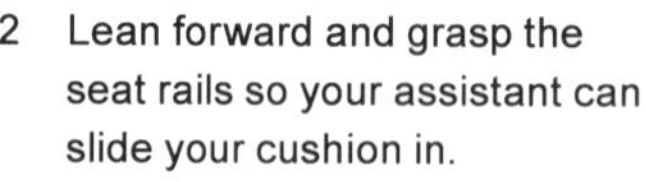

2 Lean forward and grasp the seat rails so your assistant can slide your cushion in.

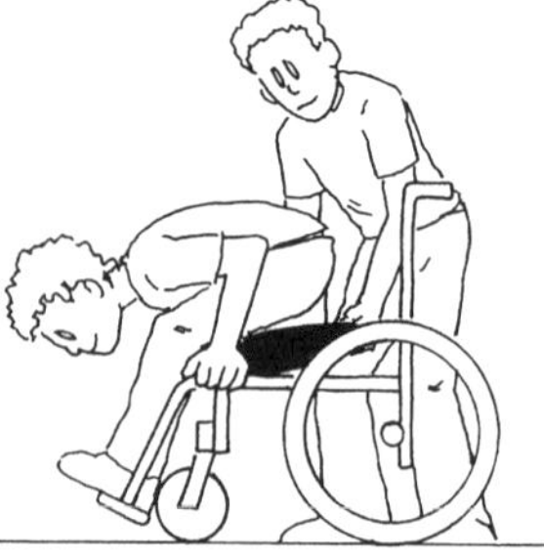

- Adjust yourself into a comfortable and stable position, with your feet on the foot supports.
- While you grasp the seat rails and lean forward, have your assistant slide your cushion back onto the seat beneath you.

With you pushing down

- Rotate the caster wheels until they are trailing forward.
- Engage your wheel locks.
- Have your assistant kneel to one side of you.
- Sit on your seat cushion at an angle to your wheelchair.
- Grab the frame on the far side of your wheelchair just in front of the seat support surface of your wheelchair.
- Put your other hand on your assistant's knee.
- On your count of three, push yourself up and into the seat of your wheelchair.
- Adjust yourself into a sitting position
- While you grasp the seat rails and lean forward, have your assistant slide your cushion back onto the seat beneath you.

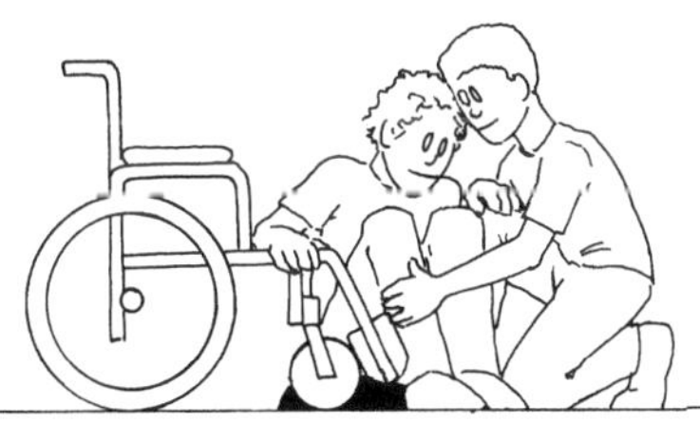

1. Have your assistant kneel at your side. Grasp the frame of the wheelchair just in front of the seat support surface of your wheelchair while sitting on your cushion.

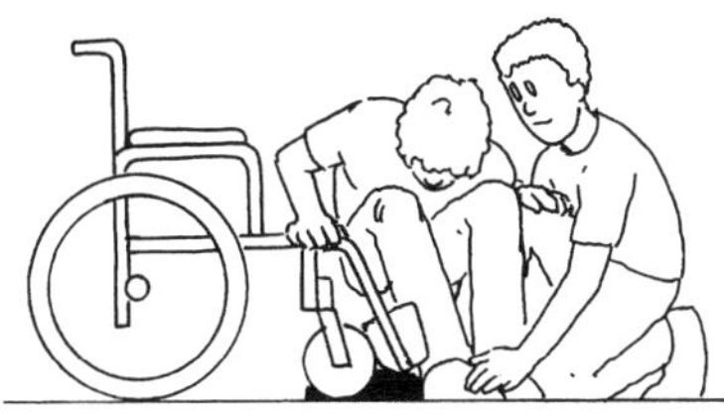

2. Use your other hand to push down on your assistant's knee.

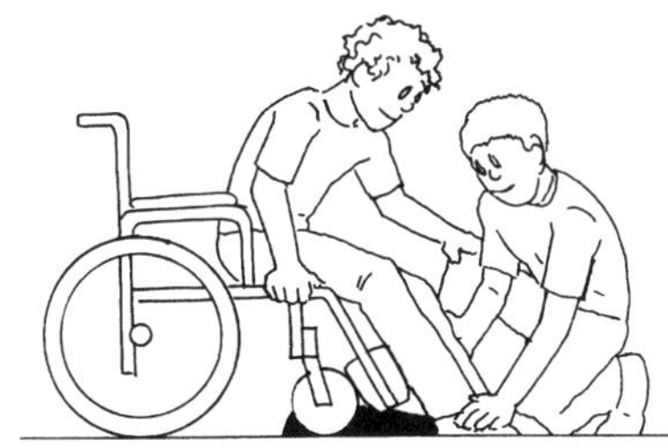

3. Continue pushing up until you are seated back in your wheelchair.

Tipping your wheelchair

- If you have fallen near your wheelchair, your assistant can tip your wheelchair over backwards so the push handles or back posts are on the ground and the foot supports are up in the air.
- With the assistant's help slide yourself back in your tipped-up wheelchair.
- Grip the handrims with your hands as your assistant kneels behind your wheelchair with their hands on the push handles or back posts.
- On your count of three, have your assistant tip your wheelchair upright while keeping his or her back as close to vertical as possible. You can help by pulling back on the handrims. Make sure you do not lose your balance forward as you come back down on all four wheels. Your assistant can place an arm across your chest to keep you from falling forward.

After getting yourself back into the wheelchair lying on its back, your assistant can tilt you upright again.

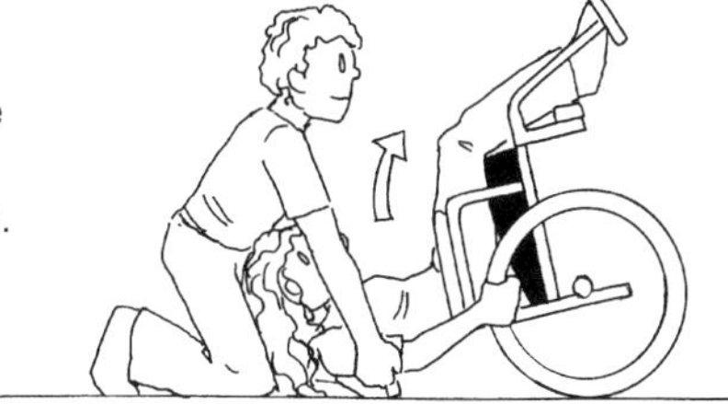

Piggyback carry

If your assistant has good leg strength and no neck or shoulder problems, he or she might be able to carry you back to your wheelchair after a fall.

- Be sure your caster wheels are trailing forward and lock your wheel locks.
- If space allows, set up your wheelchair near your body to reduce the distance your assistant must carry you.
- Sit upright on the floor with your legs spread in a wide V.
- Have your assistant squat between your legs facing away from you.
- Drape your arms around the assistant's neck, and clasp your hands together tightly.
- Have your assistant grasp your forearms.
- On your count of three, have your assistant tip forward and stand upright, keeping his or her back as straight as possible.
- Have your assistant walk to your wheelchair and bend at the knees to set you back into your wheelchair seat.

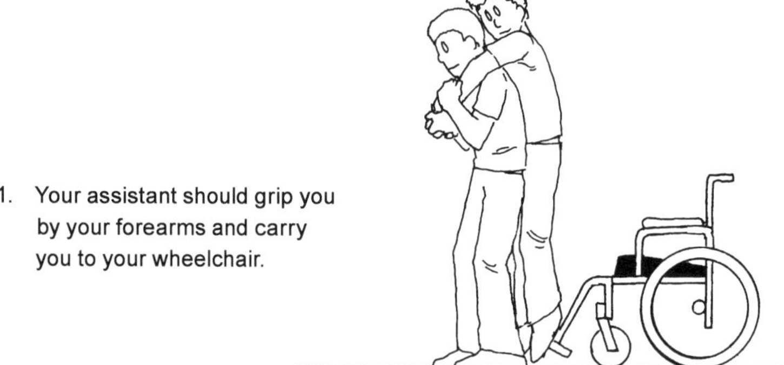

1. Your assistant should grip you by your forearms and carry you to your wheelchair.

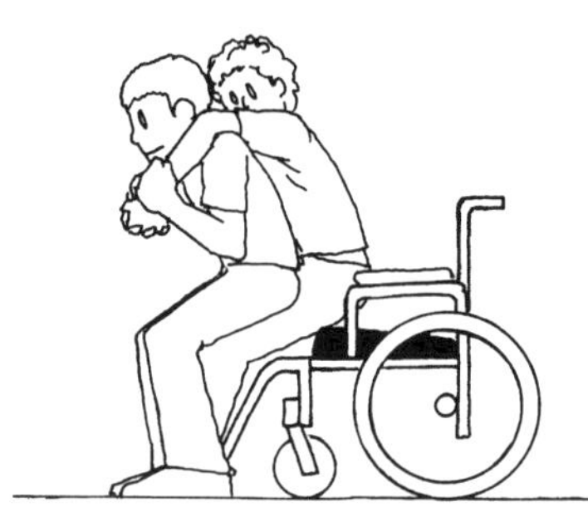

2 Your assistant should bend at the knees to set you back into your wheelchair.

Fireman's carry

- Be sure your caster wheels are trailing forward and lock your wheel locks.
- If space allows, set up your wheelchair near your body to reduce the distance your assistant must carry you.
- Wrap your arms around your assistant's neck.
- Have your assistant cradle you around the back with one arm and grasp you under the knees with the other.
- On your count of three, have your assistant lift you straight up.
- From this position, he or she can walk to your wheelchair and place you back into the seat of your chair.
- Ask your assistant to lift you using their legs, not their back muscles.

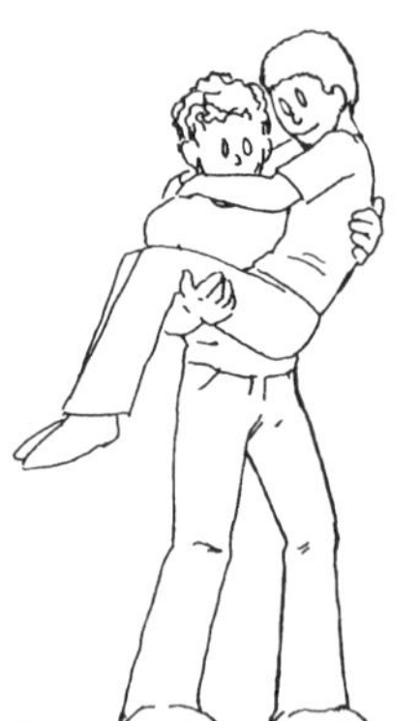

If your assistant is strong, he or she can lift and place you back into your wheelchair using a fireman's carry.

With an assistant on each side

- Be sure your caster wheels are trailing forward and your wheel locks are engaged.
- If space allows, set up your wheelchair near your body to reduce the distance your assistants must carry you.
- Have your assistants stand on either side of you, facing each other.
- Put an arm behind each person's shoulder as your assistants lock arms around your back and under your knees.
- On your count of three, both assistants should lift you up and move you over into your wheelchair.

Two assistants can form a seat with their arms to lift and carry you back to your wheelchair.

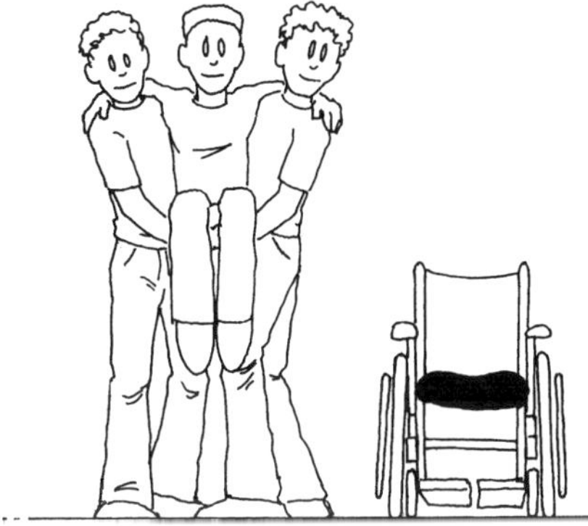

With an assistant at your head and at your feet

- Be sure your caster wheels are trailing forward and lock your wheel locks.
- If space allows, set up your wheelchair near your body to reduce the distance your assistants must carry you.
- Cross your arms in front of you.
- Have one assistant stand behind you, reaching under your crossed arms to grab and hold onto your wrists.
- Have the second assistant stand in front of you and reach forward under your legs to support your knees and/or feet.
- On your count of three, both assistants should lift you up and move you above your wheelchair seat.
- Have your assistants bend at the knees to place you in your wheelchair.

1. Have one assistant reach under your crossed arms to grasp and hold your wrists, while the other holds you under the knees.

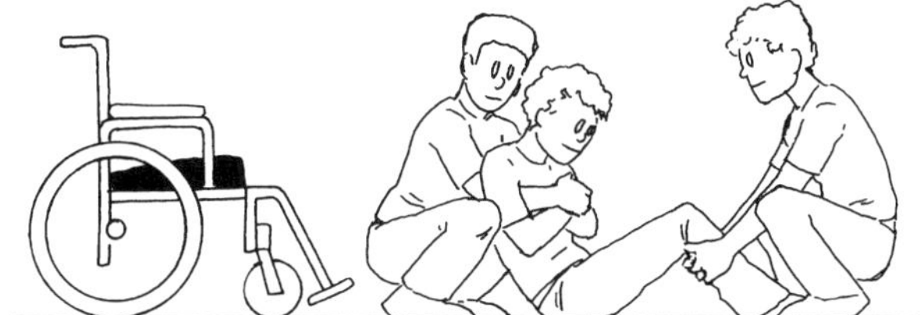

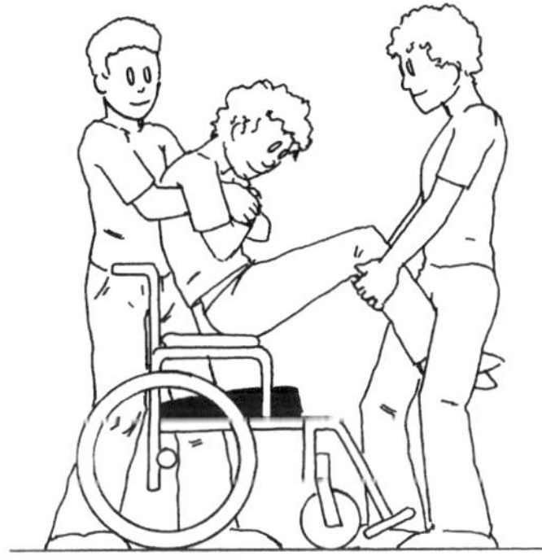

2. When you are ready, have your assistants lift and carry you over your wheelchair seat.

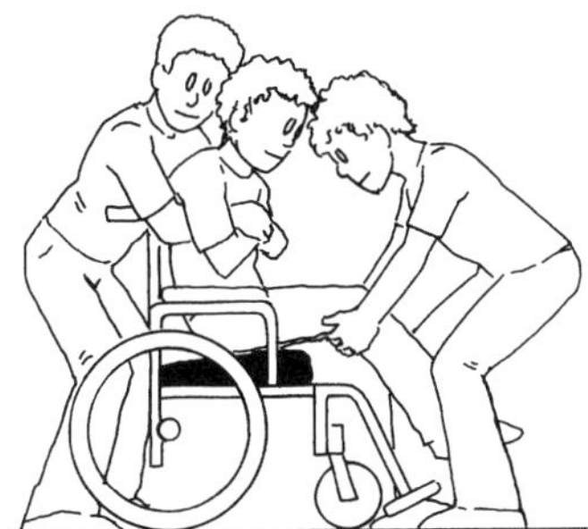

3. Your assistants should bend at the knees to place you in the chair while keeping their backs as vertical as possible.

Section 3.2

Evacuation Procedures

Carry your cell phone with you and keep it in a place that is easy for you to reach so that you can call someone if and when you need help. Consider programming a preferred assistant and emergency numbers on speed dial. If your phone has voice dialing consider using this feature in an emergency too. It is a good idea to have an emergency evacuation plan for your home, workplace, school, or other places where you spend a lot of time. Make sure your smoke detectors are working and you can reach a fire extinguisher and fire alarm pull. Find out what the safety and evacuation plan is at your apartment building, school, or work. Know what to do and where to go during each emergency situation (e.g. earthquake, tornado, fire). Know the evacuation route at your home, school, and work. Have an alternate route planned as well.

A formal evacuation plan for wheelchair users that does not require an elevator should be established for buildings with more than one level. Learn the recommended evacuation plan. In some places this might mean using a stair evacuation device, a device that attaches to a wheelchair, or a device you need to transfer into, which enables the negotiation of stairs. If a stair evacuation device is not available, consider asking a coworker or friend to carry you out of the building.

If you spend a significant amount of time on an upper floor of a building with an elevator, notify the building management and the fire department so they are aware that you are working on an upper level in the building. Find out what they recommend as the safest method to exit the building in an emergency.

Designate assistants (e.g., family members, roommates, coworkers, classmates, teachers) who are willing to help you in an emergency. Relying on other people could be a problem because they may not always be available. Practice the preferred evacuation procedure with your assistants. Be sure they know how to maneuver your wheelchair if you are unable to do so yourself, as well as how to carry you safely if you cannot evacuate in your wheelchair. Your assistants can use a blanket or curtain as a cradle to carry you down the stairs if necessary.

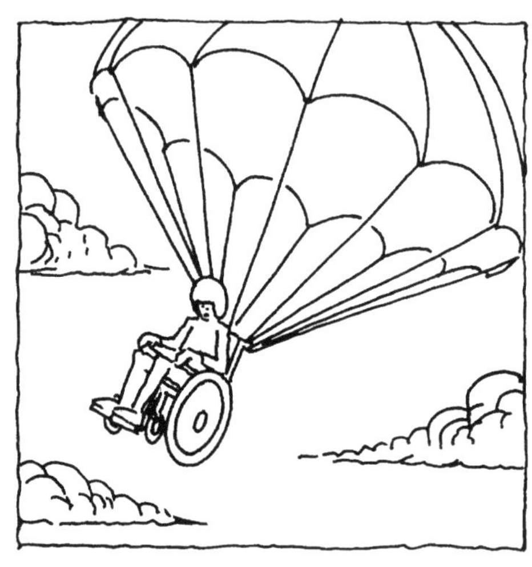

You will probably spend a lot of time out of your wheelchair at home. It may be easiest to be evacuated from your home separate from your wheelchair. Teach family members, attendants, friends, and/or roommates how to get you in and out of your wheelchair for a quick evacuation. Designate a meeting area outside your home. Be sure your neighbors know you use a wheelchair. Be sure that your local fire department knows that you use a wheelchair for your mobility as this information will be helpful for rescuers.

You should supply your local police and fire departments with a floor plan of your home and the typical sleeping location of anyone with a mobility impairment, so they can easily find you in the event of a fire or emergency evacuation.

Creating an Emergency Plan

- Designate someone in your family and someone in another geographic location as an emergency contact and keep their phone numbers handy.
- If you are separated from the people you live or work with, use your emergency contacts as an emergency headquarters to call into for help. Keep a first-aid kit available. You may want to include information about your medical condition and a list of your physician(s) and medication(s), as well as a tire pump, a flashlight, and other medical supplies.
- Take a first aid course.
- Take a CPR course.
- Take a self-defense course.
- You should have an evacuation plan for where you work, your school, your recreation facility, and at home.
- It is a good idea to actually practice your evacuation plan at least 1 time/year. When you change the clocks for daylight savings is a good day to actually perform the plan with those you have arranged to assist you in the event of an emergency. Just like running a fire drill at school or work. Practice makes perfect.

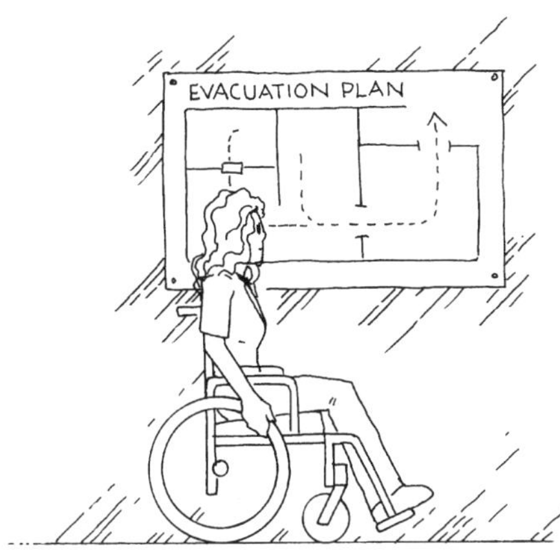

Evacuation plans should be available at work, schools, recreation facilities, and even at home.

Personal Emergency

Make sure others know about your medical conditions and can recognize the symptoms of conditions such as autonomic dysreflexia or allergies. Keep your treatment information available in case you have a medical emergency. Train those around you in emergency care techniques such as elevating your feet if your blood pressure drops or transferring you to the floor for emergency rescue purposes.

If you have a personal emergency and need to be taken to a hospital, emergency medical personnel find the following helpful:

- list of current medications and dosages
- current supply of medications in a labeled container from a pharmacy (check expiration dates)
- Medic Alert bracelet listing allergies, specific conditions and/or medications required

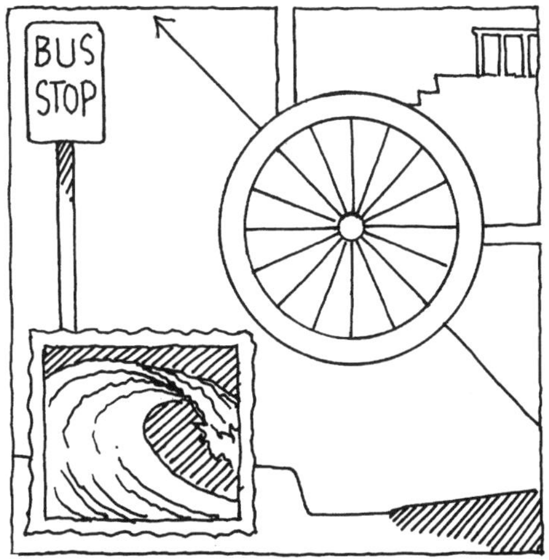

Chapter 4

Sections in This Chapter

Special Circumstances

As you become familiar with using your wheelchair, you might want to use it in circumstances other than the controlled environments previously described. This chapter addresses some of those situations. You will likely discover other useful techniques on your own.

Read the warning on page vi to learn about the risks involved in performing wheelchair skills. Falling is an unacceptable option for some wheelchair users that may result in severe injury or death.

Section 4.1

Planning Your Route

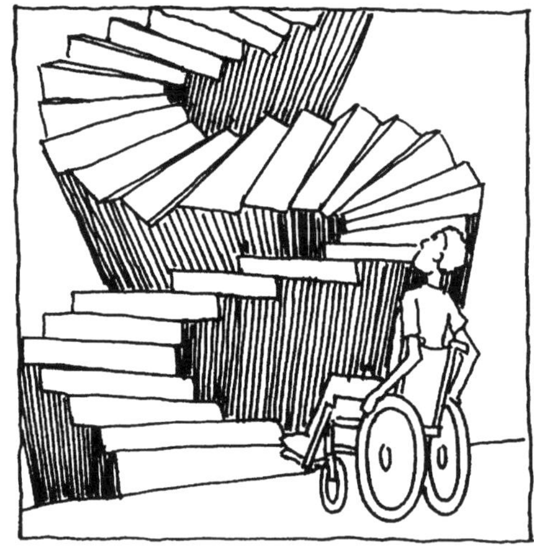

Pilots file flight plans that specify where the plane will be flying and when it is supposed to land. When planes do not arrive at their stated destinations, search parties know where to start looking. You can file a "flight plan" for your own trip. You might not be used to informing others of your travel plans, but you should do so because you are using a mechanical device that can break down. Help will arrive more quickly if someone knows where you were going.

Transit Stops

- Is there a route to transit stops that is free of curbs or stairs?
- Are there ramps or elevators from the parking area or sidewalk to the transit station and loading area?
- What is the transit stop surface made of? Can you roll across it easily or will you get stuck?
- How big is the loading area?
- Is there a shelter that can accommodate you?
- Is the stop at the other end of your route accessible? Ask these same questions about your destination stop.

Planes, Trains, and Automobiles

- Can you board the vehicle without having to transfer out of your chair? For example, are there lifts for the bus, a drop-off or rise to board a train, or a ramp or jetway to the aircraft rather than boarding stairs?
- Are there appropriate wheelchair tiedown areas, or will you have to transfer to a seat? If you do have to transfer, you will still need to make sure your wheelchair is secured or safely stored.
- Does the transit district offer lift-equipped vehicles for people with disabilities?
- Are all vehicles on the route wheelchair accessible? Find out when and where you can catch an accessible vehicle.

Rental Vehicles

- What features in your personal vehicle would you need in a rental? Most car rental companies in the United States have hand controls that can be added to any car.
- If possible, make reservations for an accessible vehicle well in advance of your trip. Most companies require at least 48 hours of advance notice to install adaptive driving equipment.
- If you are being transported in a van, ask if the vehicle has wheelchair tiedown areas or whether you have to transfer to a seat.
- Reconfirm your vehicle reservation just prior to your departure.

New Environments

Your capabilities will vary depending on your environment. For example, wheeling around a rural Midwestern town is very different from slipping through the throngs of New York City. Many factors affect wheelchair mobility, including the upkeep of sidewalks and streets.

Section 4.2

Crossing Streets

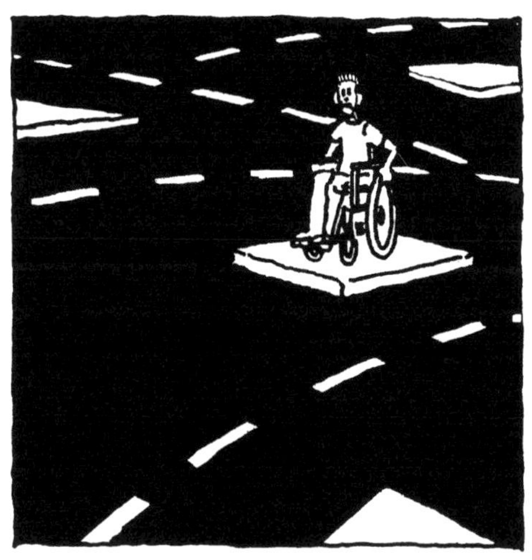

When you cross streets, watch for motorized vehicles, bicycles, and other pedestrians. Try to use a crosswalk, but remember that many motorists are unaccustomed to looking for pedestrians below eye level and drivers often ignore crosswalks without traffic lights. Be extra cautious at intersections where cars can turn right on a red light.

Before practicing the skills in this chapter, you should be able to propel a wheelchair forward and backward, at least at walking speed, cross obstacles and rough terrain, and travel up and down curb ramps and curbs.

Read the warning on page vi to learn about the risks involved in performing wheelchair skills. Falling is an unacceptable option for some wheelchair users that may result in severe injury or death.

Always use a spotter or ask someone for help if you feel uncomfortable crossing a particular street. Ask your spotter to walk next to you as you cross the street. He or she will be taller and thus more visible to motorists. A spotter can also help you maintain your balance if you have difficulty with your trunk stability.

Understand the Local Driver Mentality

In some places, motorists are more aggressive and less likely to stop for pedestrians. If you are a local resident, you will probably already be familiar with the prevailing driver mentality. If you are visiting an area for the first time, spend a few moments observing interactions between motorists and pedestrians. You may also want to ask other pedestrians about their experiences with local drivers.

Examining Street Terrain

Study the conditions of the street before you cross.

- Are there drainage grates?
- Is the road well paved or does it have potholes or bumpy surfaces?
- Are reflectors embedded in the asphalt?

- Is the surface wet or icy?
- If you do not want to go over obstacles, is there enough room to maneuver around them?

Crossing at a Crosswalk

- Always try to cross at a traffic light. Be extra cautious if there is no traffic light.
- If there is a light, try timing the street crossing interval to see if you can make it to the other side before the light changes.
- Look both ways before crossing the street. In some countries, such as England and Japan, cars drive on the left side of the road. Be especially wary when crossing streets in these places because you might forget which way to look first.

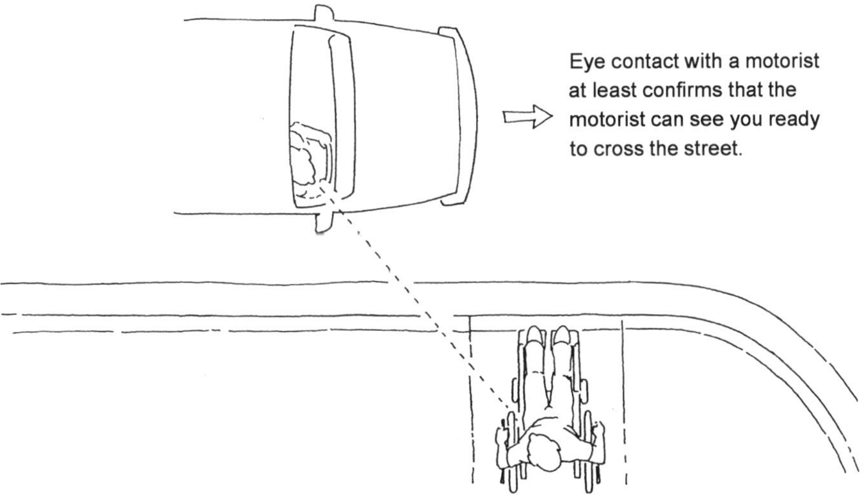

Eye contact with a motorist at least confirms that the motorist can see you ready to cross the street.

- Check for vehicles, bicyclists, or others turning right at red lights, as well as other pedestrians. Watch for turning vehicles even when crossing one-way streets, as some states permit drivers on a one-way street to turn left on a red light into another one-way street.
- Look both ways, even on one-way streets because pedestrians and some bicyclists move against traffic.
- Determine how you will move from the sidewalk to the street. Is there a curb ramp? If so, how can you best approach it? If not, can you descend the curb by yourself?
- Plan how best to ascend the curb to the sidewalk on the other side of the street. Is there a curb ramp, or will you need to climb the curb?
- Is there a center median? If so, is the surface cut through to permit you to wait in the protected area? If the median has not been cut through, is there a safe space around it for you to wait for a signal change?
- Once in the crosswalk, establish yourself by making eye contact with motorists and cyclists and edge forward so motorists know you intend to cross the street.
- Wait until all vehicles have recognized your presence and have stopped to let you cross.
- As you cross the street, keep your eyes focused on the oncoming traffic to establish eye contact with the drivers.

Crossing with No Crosswalk

- Avoid crossing between two parked cars. This is not only dangerous because passing traffic may not be able to see you, but it is also illegal!

- Some smaller intersections do not have marked crosswalks. In these instances, behave as though there were a crosswalk, but proceed with extra caution.

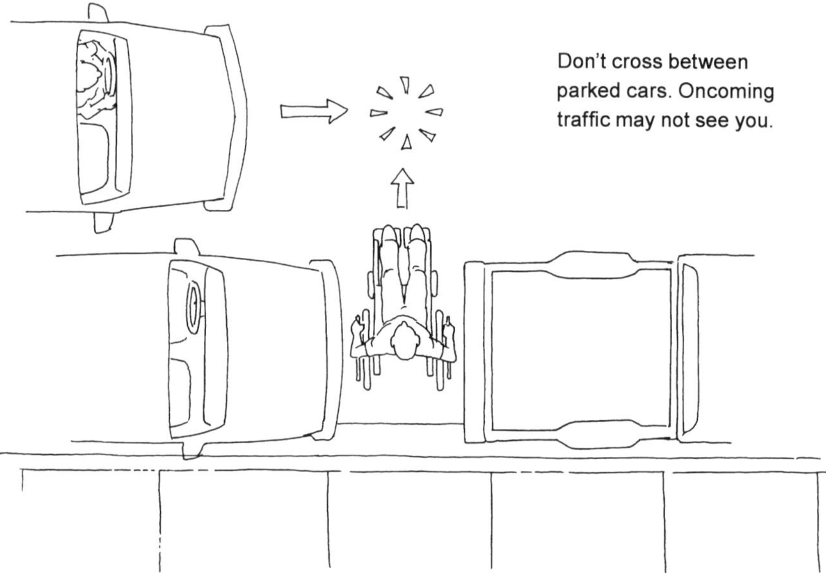
Don't cross between parked cars. Oncoming traffic may not see you.

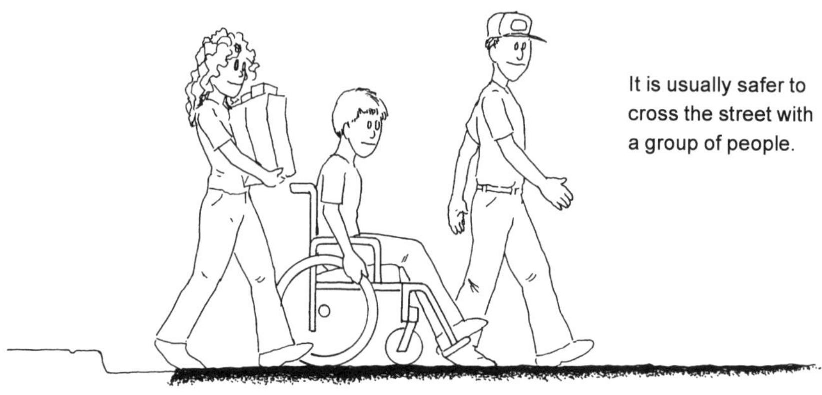
It is usually safer to cross the street with a group of people.

How to ask for assistance

If a road is busy and/or it is apparent motorists are failing to notice you, try asking for assistance.

- Look for another group crossing the street and move with them, or ask another pedestrian to walk with you as you cross.
- A group of people will be more visible to motorists, bicycles, and other pedestrians.
- Be sure to use caution. There may be safety in numbers, but you should still be aware of traffic.
- Accessories such as flags, reflectors, bright clothing, and noisemakers can improve your visibility to motorists.

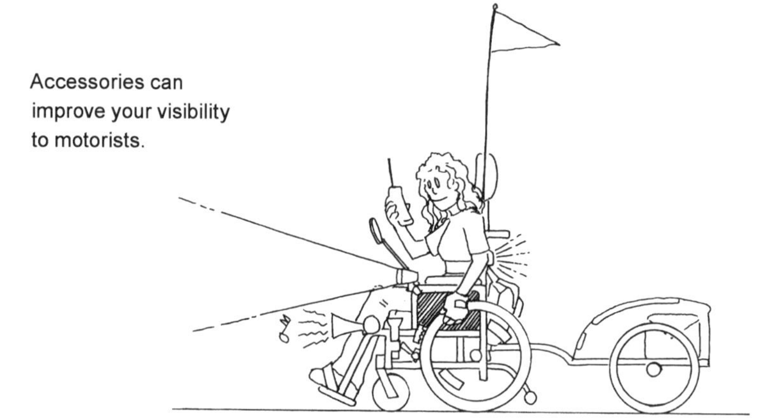
Accessories can improve your visibility to motorists.

How a spotter can help

- Walk next to the wheelchair user while crossing the street.
- Keep yourself and the wheelchair user visible to motorists.
- Prevent the wheelchair user from falling forward if the casters hit an obstacle.

Section 4.3

Nighttime Safety

While you should always be concerned with maintaining your visibility and personal safety, you should take extra precautions when traveling at night. Darkness makes everyone more vulnerable to traffic accidents as well as crime. This does not mean you should never go out after dark because every hedge hides a mugger. It does mean you should compensate for low visibility conditions and pay attention to the fact that it will be hard to see sidewalk obstructions in the dark. Stay aware of your surroundings, and make it a habit to bring safety equipment along wherever you go. A headlamp will allow you to watch the sidewalk surface in front of you so you can more safely negotiate a less than perfect sidewalk or street crossing.

Avoid potentially hazardous situations such as intersections that do not have traffic signals and unlit streets. In a wheelchair, you cannot jump out of the path of an oncoming vehicle as quickly as someone walking might be able to. Remember that even though pedestrians have the right of way in a crosswalk, many walking pedestrians are injured and killed by motor vehicles every day in pedestrian crosswalks. Be especially safety conscious when crossing streets that do not have signalized intersections and where traffic is moving at high speeds. At an intersection with a signal, make sure the traffic is stopping for the red light before going out in to the intersection as well.

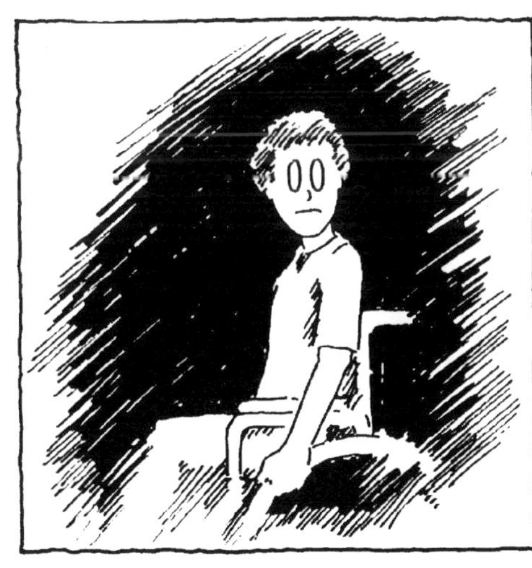

General Pointers

Increasing your visibility to others is of prime consideration when traveling at night. While you should not feel obligated to add reflectors or reflective tape to something as personal as your wheelchair, consider donning clothing or shoes made with reflective material. Running shoes and clothing commonly feature reflective strips or panels.

- Consider your path of travel. Is it safe and well lit? If not, can you take an alternate route?
- When crossing streets, make sure that you are crossing in the cross walk where motorists expect pedestrians to be. Always cross when the traffic lights indicate that it is your turn to cross. Cross in a group with other pedestrians when possible.

- Make sure someone knows you are going out and where you are going. If you are traveling and will be going out alone, inform the hotel concierge or front desk of your plans and when you expect to be back.
- Call your destination to let your friends know you are on your way and when you expect to arrive.

Visibility

Like all other pedestrians, make sure you are visible to motorists, bicyclists, and other pedestrians when you are out at night.

- Even though your wheelchair, when crossing the street, may be more visible to motorists than most ambulatory pedestrians, consider wearing light colored clothing. If you want to be more visible than other pedestrians, you should consider putting reflective tape or bicycle reflectors on your wheels or wear a lightweight or reflective jacket.

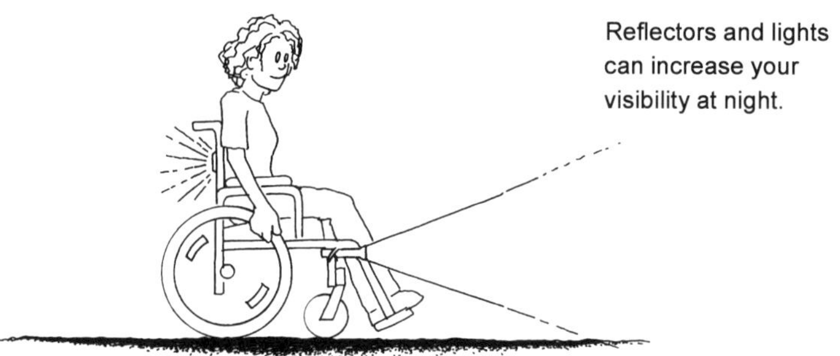

Reflectors and lights can increase your visibility at night.

- **If you intend to operative your wheelchair in a bike lane moving with or against motor vehicle traffic it is imperative that you realize that you are now operating your wheelchair like a bicycle and to maximize your safety you must reflectorize and light your wheelchair just like a bicycle.** This would mean installing reflectors on your spokes, reflectors front and rear and a white light in the front and a red light in the rear. Most bicycle lights now use LEDs and can be put into a flashing mode. A local bicycle shop can help you with adding reflectors and lighting if you intend to operate your wheelchair in this manner. Beware that your wheelchair does not have the maneuverability of a bicycle and cannot just swerve off the side of the roadway like a bicycle can. Therefore, operating your wheelchair like a bicycle in the roadway environment is extremely risky and dangerous.

Emergency Equipment

Always be prepared for emergencies. You don't need to bring a police dog, flares, and your entire set of socket wrenches; just a few essentials are indispensable in most emergencies:

- Cell phone
- Flashlight or head lamp
- Patch kit/tire pump
- Whistle or other noisemaker to attract attention
- Pepper spray

Protect Yourself

Take a self-defense course. People might pick on you, even though, and perhaps because, you use a wheelchair. Make sure the class includes verbal as well as physical self-defense. Some courses are designed specifically for women, while others are geared toward people with disabilities. Some classes specifically address the use of mace and/or pepper sprays. If your community doesn't offer a course of interest to you, ask the local Department of Recreation to offer a course or to refer you to another resource.

Moving Around

Sidewalks

- Stay on well-lit sidewalks so you can see obstacles.

Streets

- If there is no sidewalk find another route, even if it means a much longer route. It is not worth risking your life to save time. If you cannot find another route consider calling a taxi or a friend to obtain a ride.
- Beware that operating your wheelchair like a bicycle in the roadway environment is extremely risky and dangerous.
- If you decide to operate your wheelchair in the bike lane, beware that your wheelchair does not have the maneuverability of a bicycle and cannot just swerve off the side of the roadway like a bicycle can.
- The bike lane often has severe side slopes as well.
- If you do decide to operate your wheelchair in the bike lane, follow the instructions above to add reflectors and lighting to your wheelchair and move against traffic flow to monitor oncoming cars.
- Watch for parked cars with occupants, as they may not see you approach and may open a door into your path of travel.

Curbs

- Try to climb curbs only where there is enough light so you can see obstacles more easily.

Parking

- Try to park in well-lit areas.
- Make sure there is enough room to enter and exit your vehicle.
- If you parallel park your vehicle on a street, be sure your lift will unload onto the sidewalk and not into the street.

Section 4.4

Hiking

Outdoor environments can present major challenges to wheelchair navigation. Unpaved natural surfaces with soft surfaces, steep grades, and wild vegetation make trails scenic and challenging to access.

Hiking Hazards

When hiking, watch for:

- Sections of the trail that are very steep (Section 2.5 has more information about how to navigate steep slopes)
- Sections of the trail with steep side slopes (Section 2.6 has more information about side slopes)
- Soft surfaces (Section 2.4 has more information about rough terrain)
- Narrow spots on the trail (Section 2.3 has more information about navigating in tight environments)
- Obstacles such as rocks, ruts, and roots (Section 2.2 has more information about navigating over and around obstacles)

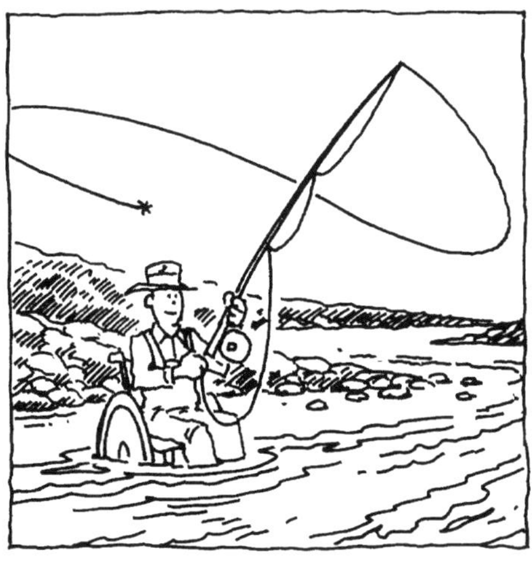

Prepare for Your Trip

Try to find out as much information as possible about a trail before you hike it. The information will help you plan a hike that meets your needs, whether you are looking for leisure enjoyment, a physical challenge, or anything else. Ask questions about:

- The length of the trail
- The average and maximum grade
- Average and maximum side slope
- Average and minimum clearance width
- Trail surface type and condition
- Trail surface firmness and stability

- Obstacles on the trail
- The best type of wheelchair setup to use (knobby tires, inner tubes, etc.)

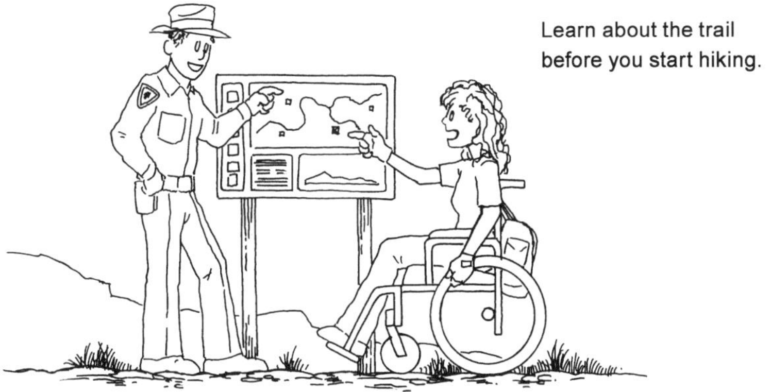

Learn about the trail before you start hiking.

Take Precautions

- Be prepared for emergencies. Carry a cellular phone, hand held "ham" radio, or other form of communication.
- Do not hike by yourself in your wheelchair. Unlike most other people, you cannot walk out if your wheelchair breaks down.

Adaptive Equipment

There are ways to modify your normal everyday wheelchair to provide enhanced mobility on hiking trails.

All terrain third wheels are available from wheelchair accessory manufacturers that can be attached to the front of your wheelchair. The attachment typically clamps onto the front of your wheelchair frame and lifts the front casters that you normally roll on up into the air. The third wheel is usually a larger diameter wheel to enable you to roll over larger obstacles and through softer surfaces.

Hiking, off road, and all terrain wheelchairs are also available that have larger wheels on all three or four wheels with lower seating to provide enhanced lateral stability. Some hiking wheelchairs have the front wheels tied together so that you can steer the wheelchair across a cross slope. Others have disk brakes which allow you to drive down slopes that are as steep as a normal flight of stairs. Others have suspension systems for flying downhill at faster speeds on logging roads after riding up ski lifts that typically take mountain bikers up the mountain in the summer.

Tow-lines can be attached to the front of any type of rehab or hiking wheelchair to enable hiking companions to assist you when needed. For everyday use, climbing slings can be purchased at a recreation equipment store. A sling that is 64 inches long made of 3/8 inch wide material will provide a loop that is 32 inches long. Wrap the sling once around the frame of your wheelchair near your knees or front casters and loop the sling through itself so that it pulls tight around your wheelchair frame.

It should be noted that there is an exception to the United States Federal Wilderness Act that allows wheelchairs, that are "suitable for use indoors", on hiking trails within these specially designated areas. Normally any wheeled device is not allowed into Federal lands designated as Wilderness Areas. This means that anything that you might take into the lobby of a hotel without getting kicked out would be acceptable. This also means that anything with an internal combustion engine would not be acceptable.

Asking for Assistance

You may need assistance from others if you encounter difficult spots along your hike.

Narrow sections with drop-offs

- Ask your spotter to walk on the downslope side of the trail.
- You may want your spotter to hold on to your chair as you travel through narrow sections of the trail.

Rocks, ruts, roots, and other obstacles

- Ask your spotter to support your chair from the side or rear while you are attempting to cross obstacles.
- Your spotter can help you cross an obstacle by pushing down and forward on the push handles to unweight the caster wheels or by pulling up and forward on the front of your wheelchair with a tow line, climbing sling or rope.
- Experiment with different attachment points to find a spot where a tow line will unweight your front caster wheels. If the attachment point is too low, the towing force will lift the front of the chair too high and could flip you over backward. If the line is too high it will tend to push your front casters even deeper into a soft surface.

Have your spotter walk along the downslope side of the trail.

Going Up and Down Hills

- Carry one or two pieces of strong rope or webbing to enable an assistant to help pull you forward or to help keep you going straight on a cross slope.
- You can attach a sling on each side of your chair to enable two people to assist you if you need more help. Having two slings will also allow your helper to always pull on the uphill side of the trail to keep you from veering in the direction of the cross slope.
- On a hiking trail, a longer sling will enable an assistant to pull further out in front of you if the trail is narrow.
- If a companion is helping you slow your descent on steep sections of the trail, use a spotter strap attached to the rear of your wheelchair as described and explained in Section 1.9 Wheelies.

Attachment of a tow line or sling at the right location on your wheelchair frame will allow an assistant to provide forward assistance and will help lift the front casters up and over obstacles.

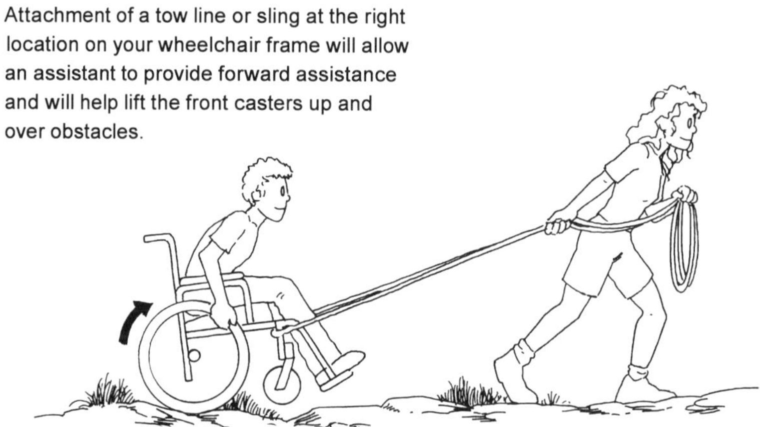

Section 4.5

Traveling

Have you ever looked forward to a fabulous meal at a great restaurant, dressed in your best clothes, and fought your way onto the bus, or endured a heart-stopping cab ride, only to find that your destination is located up a flight of stairs? Sometimes it is not a lack of access but a lack of information that will make your journey difficult. Taking a few minutes to call ahead can solve problems and save lots of time. Be specific when asking questions; many people's idea of "accessible" may be very different from yours. Do not be surprised if you are told a restaurant is accessible even if it occupies the upper floor of a building without an elevator. If a destination you have been told is accessible turns out to be inaccessible, ask to speak with the manager. Tell the manager that "accessible" means an environment in compliance with the Americans with Disabilities Act Accessibility Guidelines (ADAAG), and that your inability to use the facility probably indicates the establishment needs to improve its access measures. (Appendix A contains more information about the ADA).

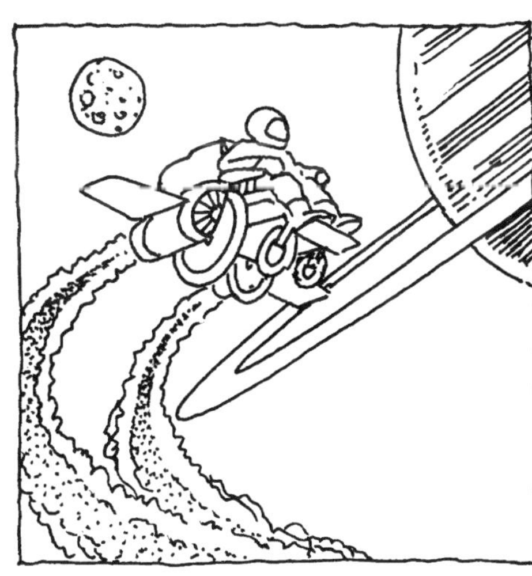

Travel Planning Tips

Part of the appeal of going to new places is the fun of exploring the unknown. Though you may think advance reconnaissance is cheating and dull, it is usually worthwhile to obtain basic access information about the site to avoid disappointments. You don't want to arrive at a wedding, dressed in nice clothing, only to find you must cross a muddy path to get to the reception. Nor would it be amusing to arrive at a hotel and discover the "accessible guest room" has a shower stall sized to accommodate slender children but not you

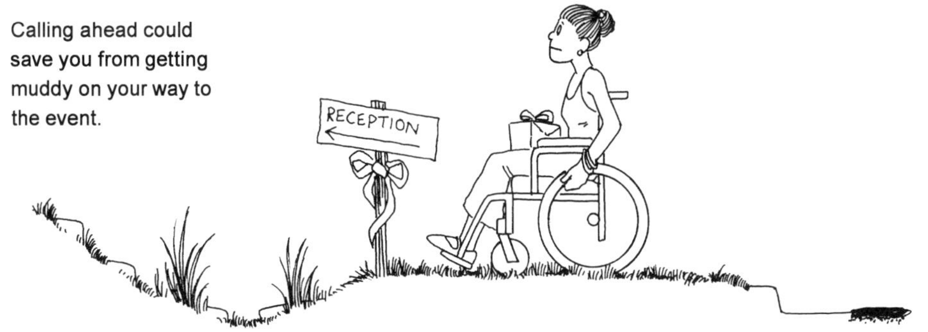

Calling ahead could save you from getting muddy on your way to the event.

and your shower chair. Make a practice of calling ahead and talking to friends or acquaintances who have been there before.

Consider asking the following questions:

- What kinds of obstacles will you face en route to your destination?
- Is there an elevator or stairs?
- Do the curbs have ramps?
- Will someone be there to help you across the lawn that's been transformed into a snow field?
- Is the route all indoors, or is a portion outdoors?
- Are there ramps or elevators leading to different levels of the destination?
- Are the elevators working?
- Are there signs to indicate the location of elevators and ramps?
- The internet gives you a brand new tool in accessibility reconnaissance – mapping sites provide a "birds eye" view that can be invaluable as a picture is worth a thousand words!

Hotel Rooms

- Is there a wheelchair accessible room? If the room is not accessible, how wide is the door leading into the room and into the bathroom?
- What floor is it on? Is there an elevator?
- What kind of knobs, handles, or latches do the doors have?
- Can you move furniture out of the way to make the room more accessible? If you do move furniture, let the housekeeping staff know that you don't want it put back in place each morning. You may also be able to arrange for the actual removal of unneeded furniture from the room.
- Can you move the bed to position your wheelchair next to it for transfers? Some hotel beds have immovable pedestals.
- Can you reach the temperature controls and drapery cords or will you need assistance?
- Is the telephone within easy reach from the bed?
- Is the TV remote control moveable or is it attached to the nightstand? If it is attached, it may be out of reach.

If your hotel room poses access problems, try brainstorming solutions with the management. For example, ask them to wrap a towel around exposed hot water pipes under sinks so you do not burn yourself, or ask maintenance to remove the bathroom door if the door itself is making the opening too narrow for your wheelchair.

Bathrooms and Restrooms

- Is the restroom on the same floor as the meeting room, or reception that you are trying to get to?
- How large is the clear-space inside of the restroom or bathroom? Is there enough space for you to turn around and get back out?
- Does the bathroom or restroom door swing into the clear-space inside the room making it impossible to get to the tub, shower or toilet?
- Can the door on a toilet stall be opened in a single swinging motion with a proper handle that you can operate with your level of hand function?
- How wide is the doorway into the toilet stall?
- Does the doorway into the toilet stall block the clear-space

needed to maneuver inside or outside of the stall? Is there a grab-bar inside for you to perform a transfer if needed?

- If the bathroom has a bathtub, does it have the clear-space adjacent to it so you can transfer into the tub and does it have grab rails needed for you to make the transfer?
- Is there a shower chair available? Most hotels have shower chairs available for your use upon request.
- If you will be transferring into a bathtub or onto a shower chair you should sit on a waterproof pressure relief cushion if you normally use a pressure relief cushion in your wheelchair. Gel cushions and small strap on cushions are available that will provide pressure relief when sitting on the edge of a bathtub, in a bathtub or on a shower bench.
- Bath towels are often high up on a shelf over the toilet. Are the towels placed within reach?

This tub would be usable if the door could close behind the wheelchair user. Calling beforehand could have prevented this situation.

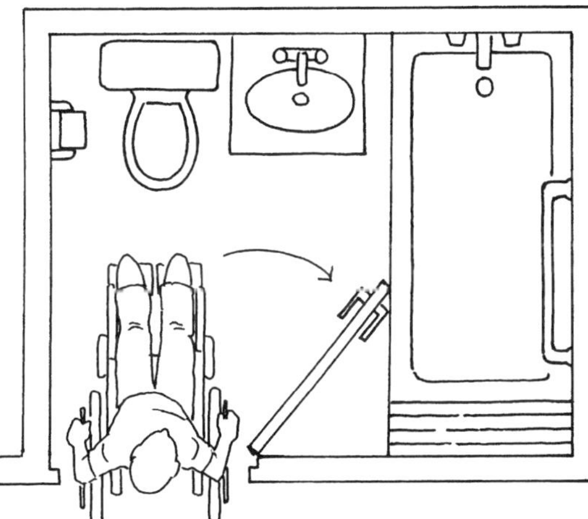

Section 4.6

Weather

Weather and the residues of weather impact your ability to use your wheelchair. For example, on a windy day you might feel your wheelchair being pushed by the wind and have to compensate to keep going straight. Depending on where you live, it might be useful to learn to negotiate snow and icy surfaces as well as rain puddles and mud.

Have a spotter walk beside your wheelchair the first few times you encounter a new weather condition. Your spotter should be ready to prevent you from falling if you lose your balance and to help you pull or push your wheelchair if you get stuck.

Consider the following before traveling in bad weather:

- Be prepared before you go outside.
- Wear the proper clothing for the weather outside.
- Be sure your tires have tread and are in good condition.
- You might want to carry a flashlight or a headlamp.
- Think about the route you plan to take to avoid steep hills if it will be icy.
- Plan a route that will not require you to cross terrain that will be difficult in the existing weather conditions.
- Determine if there is an alternative route that would be safer and/or easier.

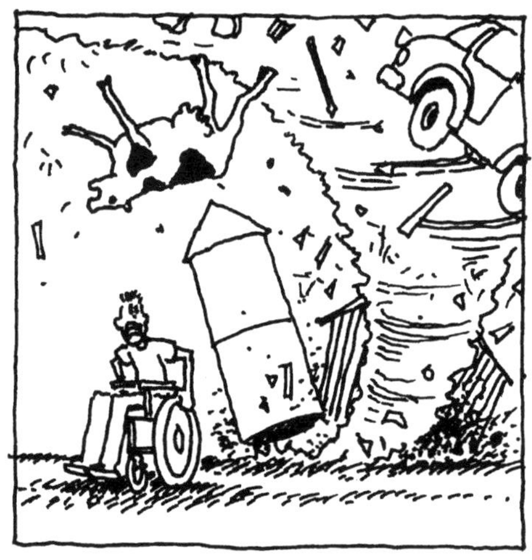

Precipitation

Stow extra rain and snow gear in places you spend a lot of time, such as your home, car or office. This way you will be prepared for a change in weather conditions. Consider using a poncho-style slicker with a hood. This versatile piece of outerwear will help keep you dry and can be positioned to cover items you need to carry on your lap. Tuck the slicker's edges under your legs to avoid catching the fabric in your wheels. Clothing guards can help protect your garments from getting splattered with water. A hat with a wide brim can prevent the rain and snow from dripping down your neck. Gloves with a grip are good for keeping your hands warm and dry.

Rain

- Look at the surface ahead of you as you move around in rainy weather.
- Be cautious of obstacles such as grates that might be hiding under puddles, particularly at curb ramps. Puddles can be deeper than they look.
- Before initiating your own crossing, observe pedestrians crossing the same area.
- Remember that some wet surfaces are slippery. Moving slowly will help you stay in control. Even if you are on a familiar surface, it will be more slippery than when it is dry.

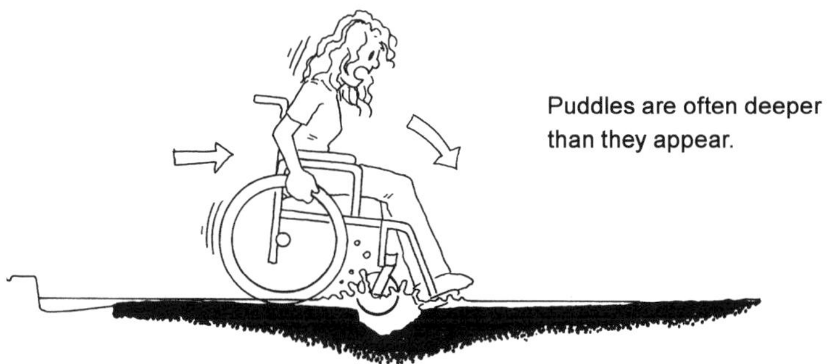

Puddles are often deeper than they appear.

Ice, snow, and slush

After a snowstorm, a familiar area may look entirely different. There may be uneven travel surfaces due to packed snow and melting ice. Passages may be narrower because of the accumulation of snow and snow banks, and hazards such as grates can be concealed under a uniform blanket of white. When approaching an intersection, your visibility and the visibility of motorists will be greatly reduced, and motorists may not see you crossing the street. Remember to allow yourself extra time to travel through the hazardous conditions.

The type of tires you use affects how you move on ice. Pneumatic and treaded tires grip surfaces better than solid or ribbed ones.

- Look at the surface ahead of you as you move around in snow, ice, or slushy weather.
- Check for icy patches and obstacles such as grates that might be hidden under snow or slush, particularly at curb ramps. Slush is often deeper than it looks. Observe pedestrians crossing the same area.
- Proceed slowly on icy surfaces.
- Slush and snow will affect you much like the rough terrain of sand and gravel. To avoid getting stuck, watch your caster wheel position when changing directions. Keep both caster wheels pointed in the same direction for maximum stability.

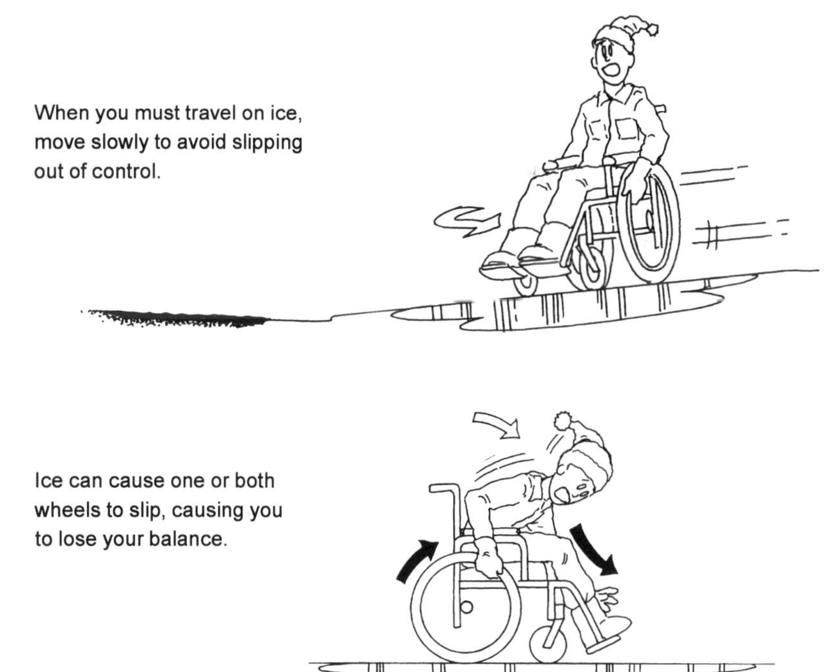

When you must travel on ice, move slowly to avoid slipping out of control.

Ice can cause one or both wheels to slip, causing you to lose your balance.

Traveling in snow with an assistant

- Since your caster wheels will sink into snow, ask an assistant to push down and forward to reduce the level of drag on them as you push forward.
- Alternatively, have someone tie a rope or a spotter strap to the front of your wheelchair to tow you. If attached correctly, the rope or webbing will pull the caster wheels up out of the snow.

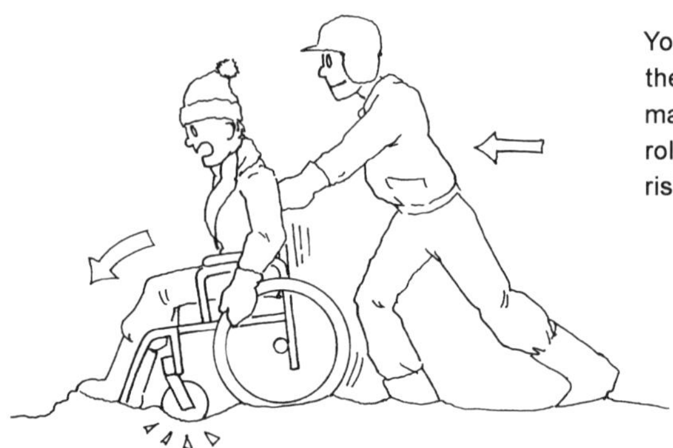

Your casters may plow into the snow instead of over it, making it difficult to continue rolling. This may put you at risk of a forward fall.

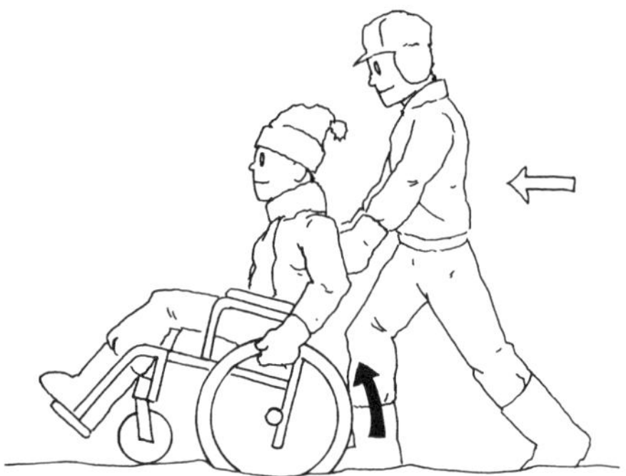

Ask your assistant to keep your wheelchair in a wheelie when traveling on snow.

Sun

If you live in a place that gets hot or humid, consider keeping loose and light clothing handy. Keep a hat in your clothing stash to shade your eyes from the sun and a sweatband or bandanna to keep the sweat out of your eyes. Sunglasses can protect your eyes from the sun and limit glare. Carry a water bottle with you at all times, especially in the summer. If your wheelchair has been stored in the sun, car trunk, or other hot area, the metal can get very hot. Be careful not to burn yourself if your sensation is impaired.

Wind

Keep long hair tied back when venturing into very windy weather. This will help keep your hair out of your eyes. Eyeglasses and sunglasses can keep dirt from blowing in your eyes.

- Look at the surface ahead of you as you move around in windy weather. Be cautious of obstacles that might have blown onto the surface.
- In strong wind, you may need to compensate to maintain a straight path.

How a spotter can help

- Walk beside the wheelchair user.
- Be ready to prevent the wheelchair user from falling forward or backward.

Section 4.7

Transportation

Your wheelchair will probably not be the only method of transportation you will use. Boarding, traveling on, and exiting other methods of transportation with your wheelchair can require special techniques and equipment to travel safely.

Cars

Most manual wheelchairs can be folded or taken apart for ease of travel, and most wheelchairs must be folded to fit into cars. If your wheelchair cannot be taken apart or folded, or if you cannot transfer safely from your wheelchair to the vehicle seat, you will need to ride in a minivan, full-size van, or other larger vehicle. If you transfer to the vehicle seat and are going to be riding a long distance and you are prone to pressure sores, use your wheelchair cushion in the vehicle seat. If your cushion is insufficient to support you comfortably, you may need to get a different cushion and back support to use when sitting in a vehicle seat. Many people who use a wheelchair have a one-inch thick gel cushion that provides some level of pressure relief when used over the contoured seating of many vehicle seats. A low-profile cushion like this will not add significantly to your sitting height if you are driving a vehicle, thereby allowing you to have a good view of the road through the windshield. If you normally travel with a small cushion in your luggage for use in the bathroom, consider sitting on this cushion for pressure relief when riding in a vehicle seat. Always use the vehicle's safety belt. A seat-belt system with a lap and shoulder belt offers the best protection should you end up in an accident. Usually, you can slightly recline the back of the vehicle seat to assist you with maintaining your balance and sitting posture.

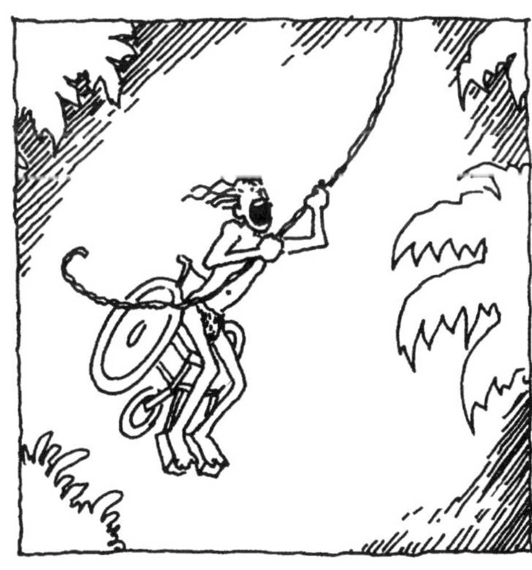

There are a few common methods to transfer into a passenger car. Two-door vehicles have larger doors that open wide, making it easier to transfer into the vehicle seat. If you will be using a 2-door car, you will want to transfer into the front seat. You can get in either from the driver or passenger's side. If you are driving but get in on the passenger's side, you will have to scoot over to the driver's seat which can be difficult in today's vehicles with bucket seats and gear-shift consoles in the center of the vehicle.

If you plan to transfer from you wheelchair to drive and you get in on the driver's side, there are several options for getting your wheelchair into the car. If your wheelchair folds to become narrow you can sometimes sit sideways with your legs outside of the car, move the driver's seat forward to increase the space behind it, and release the seat back to fold forward slightly against your back. You can then roll and lift your wheelchair into the back seat directly behind you. If you have quick-release wheels on your wheelchair, you can remove them and put them in the back seat or in the front passenger seat beside you. Then you can fold your wheelchair frame and lift it into the back seat or passenger seat beside you. Many drivers recline the back of the vehicle seat to provide more clearance before lifting their wheelchair frame in the car to place it in the front passenger seat.

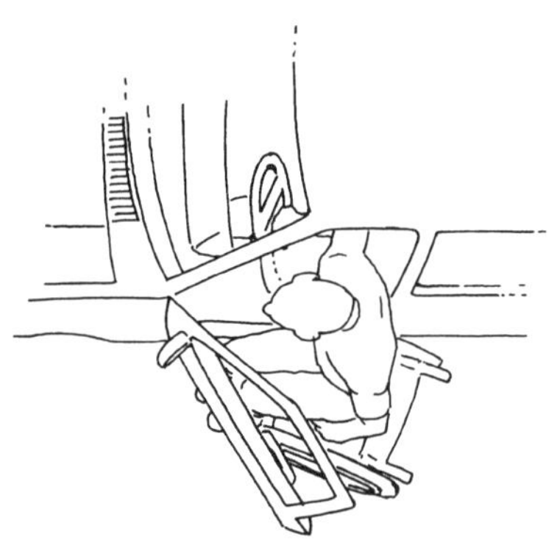

1. Open the vehicle door and pull up next to your vehicle at a slight angle.

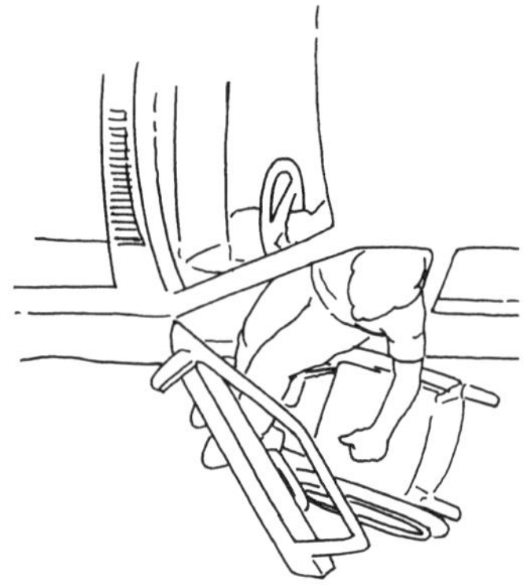

2. Transfer into the vehicle seat. The steering wheel, vehicle seat cushion, door frame, and/or wheelchair seat rails or arm supports can be used for leverage to help you transfer.

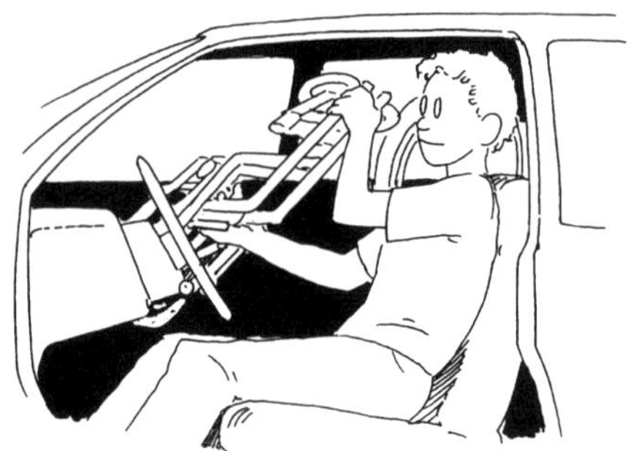

3. If your wheelchair folds, you may be able to slide it over your lap and store it on the passenger seat next to you or behind you in the back seat. It will be easier if you are able to take the rear wheels off first.

Driving

If you can get into the vehicle's driver seat but do not have leg function, your vehicle will need to be equipped with hand controls so you can operate the brake and accelerator pedals by hand. Contact a vehicle modification professional in the community or your rehab facility to get more information about adaptive-driving controls. If you are purchasing a new vehicle, be aware that many car companies have a hand-control program and will include the cost of installing hand controls with the purchase of the vehicle.

If you are unable to transfer into the seat of a standard passenger car, you can order a full-size van or minivan with a lowered floor and fold down ramp or power lift for occupied-wheelchair access into the vehicle. Full-size vans can be ordered with electrically powered platform lifts for wheelchair access into the van. Vans can be set up to drive from your wheelchair with a wheelchair lock-down system but it is always safer to transfer and drive while sitting in the vehicle manufacturer's seat. Electric tracks are available to modify the driver's seat so that it moves further back for the transfer and then moves forward to the driving position.

If you are going to rent a vehicle in the U.S., you can request a rental car with hand controls if you inform the rental-car company with at least 48 hours of advance notice. There are also portable hand controls that you can purchase and take with you in your luggage. They can be quickly installed in any vehicle with an automatic transmission. This is particularly useful if you travel with less than 48 hours notice, or if you are traveling to another country where rental cars with hand controls are not available. In some cities, rental vans with ramps or lifts with hand controls may be available.

Taxis and Paratransit Vans

Riding in a taxi should not be a problem if you use a manual wheelchair and can transfer to the front or rear seat of a 4-door sedan. You or the driver will need to fold your wheelchair and possibly remove your larger quick-release wheels so the driver can stow your wheelchair inside the vehicle or in the trunk.

Some cities have ramp or lift-equipped taxi services that allow you to remain in your wheelchair when entering the vehicle before transferring to a vehicle seat, or to remain seated in your wheelchair when traveling. Most of these taxi and paratransit companies require two or more days of advance notice for the scheduling of lift-equipped vehicles.

Electronically powered hydraulic lifts are usually available to lift you while seated in your wheelchair into the vehicle but paratransit minivan vehicles will typically provide a ramp for you to enter and exit the vehicle in your wheelchair. Personal vehicle lifts are designed to be operated by the wheelchair user, while lifts on public and paratransit vehicles are designed to be operated by the driver of the vehicle. It is always safest to back onto a platform lift when entering a vehicle and to move forward onto the lift platform when exiting the vehicle, so that you are always facing away from the vehicle. However, in vehicles with lifts at the back of the vehicle (i.e. rear entry), you will probably need to face forward and toward the vehicle while on the lift if you are going to remain in your wheelchair while traveling facing forward. In these cases, it is important that a safety belt is placed behind you before the lift moves. Also, all lifts should have a roll-stop barrier to prevent your wheelchair from rolling off of the lift platform.

If there is a vehicle seat that you can transfer into inside the vehicle you should do so for safety reasons. Using the vehicle lap-and-shoulder-belt restraints designed for that seating position is the safest way to travel. Your wheelchair can then be stored in a cargo area or secured in the vehicle.

If there is no seat to transfer into, or if you are not able to transfer to the vehicle seat easily and safely, the driver should secure your wheelchair with you sitting in it using a forward facing four-point, strap-type tiedown system. When you remain in your wheelchair for travel, your wheelchair should always be secured facing the front of the vehicle and should never be secured facing sideways or backward. If the securement system is oriented for use with side-facing wheelchairs, it has not been installed correctly and, for your own safety, you should refuse to be transported in this manner.

In addition to the wheelchair tiedown system, the wheelchair-occupant space should be provided with a lap-and-shoulder seatbelt system similar to that provided by seatbelts used by passengers sitting in vehicle seats. You should always make sure that the driver places this lap and shoulder belt on you with the lap belt positioned low on your pelvis and the shoulder belt crossing over the middle of your shoulder that is closest to the sidewall of the vehicle, with the lower end connecting to the lap belt near your hip on the opposite side. The lap-belt portion of the seatbelt should never be placed over or in front of your wheelchair's arm supports.

Touring Buses and Trains

Call ahead to purchase tickets and to determine if the touring bus has a lift. Making a reservation for a touring bus or train is a good idea. Verify if there is a wheelchair accessible train car available.

Getting on and off touring buses and trains often requires assistance if there is no lift built into the vehicle. If a lift or ramp is not available, it is usually safest and easiest to have someone help you transfer into a vehicle seat, get you positioned, and then store your wheelchair.

When the boarding platform on a train is elevated to the same height as the entrance, an assistant will usually place a bridge plate across the gap to help you roll into the car. When the boarding platform is not level with the train car, a portable ramp is usually dropped into place for you to enter. Most trains have a car with a bathroom designed for wheelchair access and a space for you to ride the train sitting in your own wheelchair. The conductors on the train and at the stations are usually helpful with handling luggage and any additional assistance you might need.

Riding in your wheelchair in a van, bus, or train

No matter what type of transportation you are taking, the safest way to travel is in the vehicle seat if the seat is facing forward and the seating position is provided with a crashworthy lap/shoulder seatbelt system. When you transfer, use the seat belts that come with the vehicle. If you need additional torso support to stay upright, you may be able to adjust the angle of the seat back rearward to help you maintain your balance.

- If the public transportation seats are not provided with seatbelts, but there is a place for you to position your wheelchair facing forward that is equipped with wheelchair tiedown straps and a lap/shoulder seatbelt system, it is better to stay in your wheelchair and use the location provided for your wheelchair.
- Make sure your wheelchair is properly secured to the vehicle floor facing forward using all four straps of a four-point tiedown system, as described in the taxi section above. A separate seatbelt system consisting of a lap and diagonal shoulder belt should be used to secure you in position. If an accident occurs, or if there is an abrupt stop, it is important that you remain in your wheelchair and that your wheelchair remains secured in place to reduce the risk of serious injuries to you and other passengers in the vehicle.
- If you customarily ride in vehicles while seated in your wheelchair, consider using a rear head support attached to your wheelchair back support to help prevent head and neck injuries in case of an accident. Car seats have rear head restraints to help prevent neck injuries in rear impacts. As a wheelchair user, you would also benefit from a head support attached to your wheelchair that is positioned at least as high as your ears and within two inches of the back of your head.
- If you are uncomfortable with the method used to secure your wheelchair or with the seatbelt system provided in the vehicle, get off the vehicle and seek an alternate form of travel. Do not put yourself at risk.

Rear-facing wheelchair passenger stations in large city buses

For some large intra-city buses that travel at relatively slow speeds it is very unlikely that the bus will be involved in a serious accident. These vehicles typically allow passengers to travel standing while holding onto hand grips for stability during starts and stops. Some of the newer low-floor intra-city buses are equipped with rear-facing wheelchair passenger stations that are designed to keep the wheelchair in position and keep you in your wheelchair during non-crash vehicle maneuvers. To use these systems you only need to be able to back your wheelchair up against a padded, rear facing forward barrier. If you do not have wheel locks, there may be a seat belt attached to the forward barrier or floor that can be used to keep you and your wheelchair from rolling backward in the vehicle during vehicle start up, or from rotating into the aisle during turns. When using a rear-facing wheelchair passenger space, it is always a good idea to use a postural lap belt attached to your wheelchair to keep you from falling out of your wheelchair during acceleration. Some wheelchair users may also be able to hold onto the large wheels or the hand rims of their manual wheelchairs to hold themselves in position. There may be a horizontal or vertical bar located in the rear-facing passenger space to hold onto. Some wheelchair stations for rear-facing ridership on a bus that are currently under development will provide a mechanism for holding your wheelchair in place by squeezing the sides of the wheelchair with soft surfaces that won't damage your equipment.

Transportable Wheelchairs

You should be aware that you can now order most manual and many power wheelchair models with a "transport option," also known as "WC19 wheelchairs." The transport option means that the wheelchair has specific locations on the chair frame that are identified for quicker, easier, and more effective securement using a four-point, strap-type tie-down system. These wheelchairs have been crash tested to verify that the wheelchair will not come apart or contribute to any injuries that you might receive in most crash situations. They also provide the user with the option of using a crash-tested wheelchair-anchored lap belt to which a vehicle shoulder belt can be connected to complete a three-point seatbelt system.

Secure your wheelchair so it
won't take any trips without you!

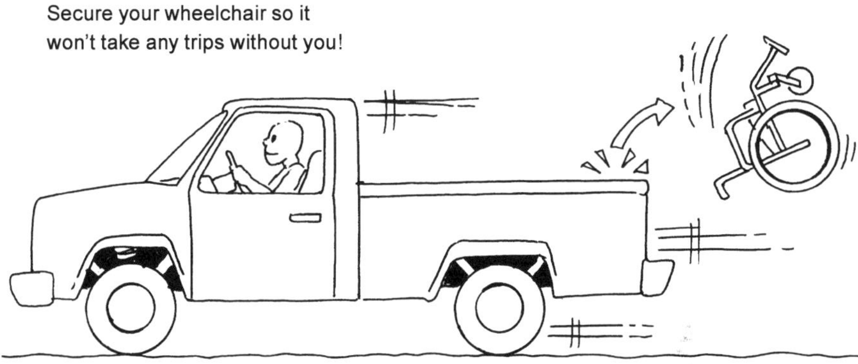

Air Travel

Reservations

When making a flight reservation online you can usually indicate that you use a wheelchair and you can indicate if you can or cannot walk to your seat. When making a seat selection, you will not be allowed to sit in an emergency exit row. If you cannot walk to your seat you will need to be assisted to your seat using an aisle chair. An aisle chair is a very narrow chair on wheels that an airport assistant can roll to bring you onto the plane and to your seat.

Some people prefer to sit in an aisle seat because it is the easiest to transfer into. Others prefer sliding over to the window seat so other passengers do not have to climb over them to go to the bathroom. Most planes do not have accessible bathrooms. On longer flights, small aisle wheelchairs are often stored in the passenger compartment that you can use with assistance to reach the bathroom. On these aircraft, the bathroom door often opens up larger and there is a curtain available so you can get close to and use the toilet.

Boarding

When you check in at the luggage counter you should request a gate check tag for your wheelchair. Be sure to carry any medical supplies that you may need during the flight. Also be sure to carry any medical supplies that you may need in a carry on in case your luggage were to be lost when you arrive at your destination.

There is usually a special line at security for wheelchair passengers. You will often be directed to a different area for screening. You will receive a separate screening that will generally take much more time than it takes for other passengers. You may generally request a private screening if you so desire. You will receive a physical pat down and your wheelchair and cushion will be screened by a person of the same sex. Plan on needing additional time compared to other passengers at the security checkpoint even though you will usually not have to wait in as long a line as other passengers.

If you arrive and check in at the gate at least 30 minutes early, you can request to pre-board the aircraft. If the aircraft has a closet and you have checked in at least 30 minutes early and you have a cross brace style folding wheelchair and you are the first wheelchair passenger to check in, then you can request to have your wheelchair stored on board the aircraft in the closet. Otherwise your wheelchair will be transported in the cargo hold and will be brought back up to the door of the aircraft when you arrive at your destination. When you check in at the gate be sure to get a wheelchair gate check tag if you did not do so when you checked in at the front counter where you checked any luggage you might have.

Most airplane aisles, especially those on commuter aircraft, will be too narrow to accommodate your wheelchair. You may be able to remove your rear wheels and roll on your anti-tip devices, or have an assistant traveling with you to hold up the back of your wheelchair and roll it down the aisle on the front caster wheels. (See Section 2.3 for more information about using your wheelchair in tight environments.) You will most likely need to transfer into an aisle chair and be moved to your seat by airport assistants. Remember to bring your wheelchair cushion or other postural support devices (PSDs) for a more comfortable plane ride and to provide pressure relief while sitting in the aisle chair and in the aircraft seating.

When it is time to pre-board the aircraft you will transfer into the aisle chair at the door of the aircraft toward the end of the jet-way. The jet-way can be steep, especially at the transition ramps between sections of the jet-way. If you cannot perform wheelies down these transition ramps you will want to turn around backwards and have the airport assistant help you back down these ramps. Your wheelchair will be folded and tagged for gate delivery at this point. It might be safer for you to carry your accessories on board, including your arm supports and foot supports so they do not become lost or damaged. If you have a folding wheelchair, you might want to use a bungee cord or Velcro™ strap to prevent it from unfolding in the cargo hold. The airport assistant will assist you with the transfer onto the aisle chair if needed and will use seat belts to keep you positioned on the aisle chair. The airport assistant will then roll the aisle chair down the aisle of the aircraft backwards to your seat. The airport assistants will then assist you with the transfer into your seat if needed. If you sit on a pressure relieving cushion, you should sit on the cushion on top of the aircraft seat.

Make sure the head flight attendant is aware that you will need your own wheelchair brought up from the cargo hold and that you will need an aisle chair to disembark from the aircraft. You will get off the aircraft last at your destination with assistance from the airport staff using the aisle chair and then getting into your wheelchair at the door of the aircraft.

If your wheelchair will fit down the aisle without the rear wheels, have your personal assistant roll you to your seat on the front casters.

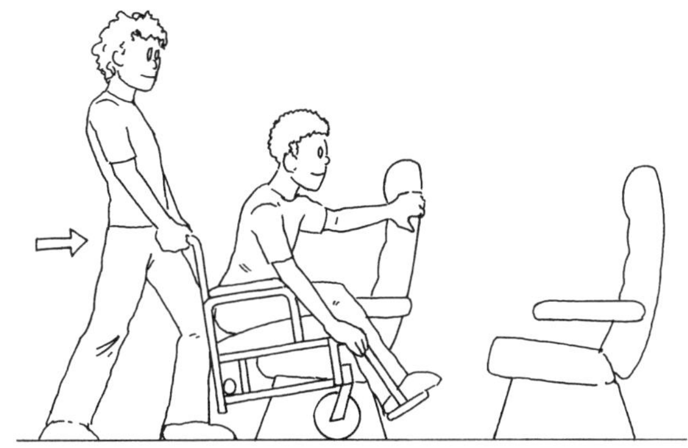

Boarding an aircraft using an aisle chair

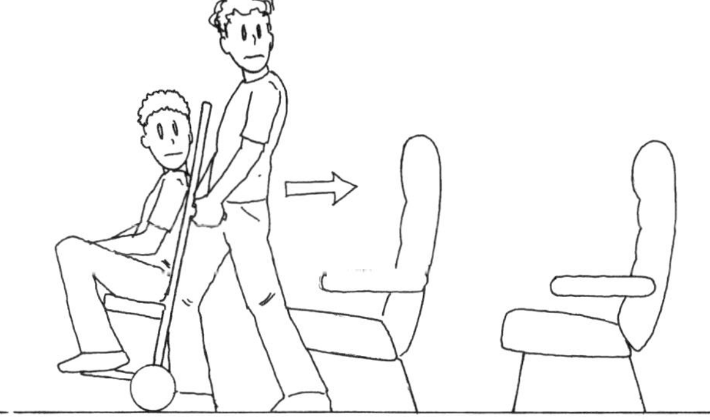

Making flight connections

When planning to make flight connections between planes, have your wheelchair tagged to be brought to the aircraft door at the transfer destination. This way you can use your own wheelchair to travel from one gate to the next. You will be getting off the aircraft after all other passengers are off the aircraft. You should plan on longer connection time between flights than required for other passengers. One hour or more would be the minimum connection time recommended between flights.

After landing

Once at your destination, make sure your wheelchair has been reassembled correctly. If anything is broken or missing, speak immediately with an air carrier representative for help. If you are worried about the handling of your mobility equipment, carry a copy of the Air Carriers Access Act regulations to help settle potential disputes. If you travel with a service dog, pack a copy of state regulations regarding service dog access. Both regulations should be available from the office of your state's Attorney General.

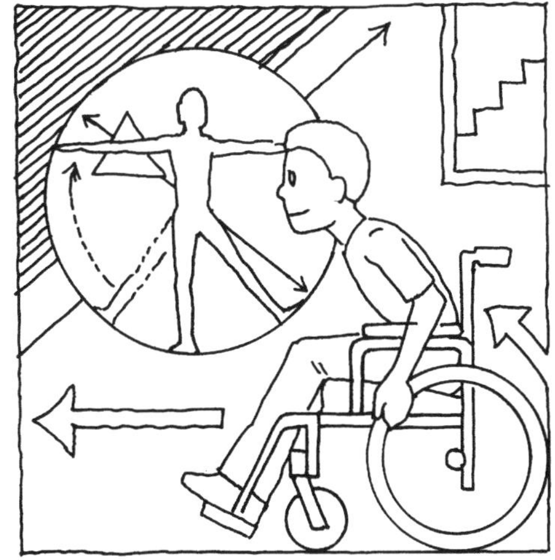

Chapter 5

Sections in This Chapter

Body Mechanics

This chapter is meant as a guide for those who assist wheelchair users. While lifting and pushing a wheelchair user might not appear as risky as playing football or moving furniture, the types of injuries that can result, can be identical. The wheelchair user should also read this chapter to help protect spotters and assistants from injury. While reading this chapter, consider circumstances that will put you at risk for injury while helping a wheelchair user. Think of better ways to handle or avoid hazardous situations.

Remember that assisting a wheelchair user could expose you to serious injury or death. Read the warning on page vi to learn more about the risks involved in performing these techniques.

Section 5.1

Protecting Yourself

"Body mechanics" is a term used to describe the positioning and use of the body. Improper body mechanics when assisting a wheelchair user can result in injury to that person or you. Common injuries include back strain and pulled muscles.

Body Position

Be aware of your body when you are assisting someone. If any part of your body hurts or feels awkward, you may not be positioned properly or you may have reached your physical limits. Stop and seek additional help.

Helping a wheelchair user can require a lot of pushing, pulling, and/or lifting. Always observe the following safe body mechanics principles to avoid straining your back.

- Bend your knees, not your waist to keep your back straight and perpendicular to the floor as much as possible.Use your legs for strength rather than the weaker muscles of your back or stomach to prevent injury.
- Use a spotter strap to prevent the wheelchair user from tipping over backwards as described and explained in Section 1.9 Wheelies.
- Do not lock your knees.
- Never twist your waist. Instead, keep your torso facing the same direction as your hips. Pivot your feet to change direction.
- Keep your back straight. Hunching over or rounding your shoulders can also cause back strain.

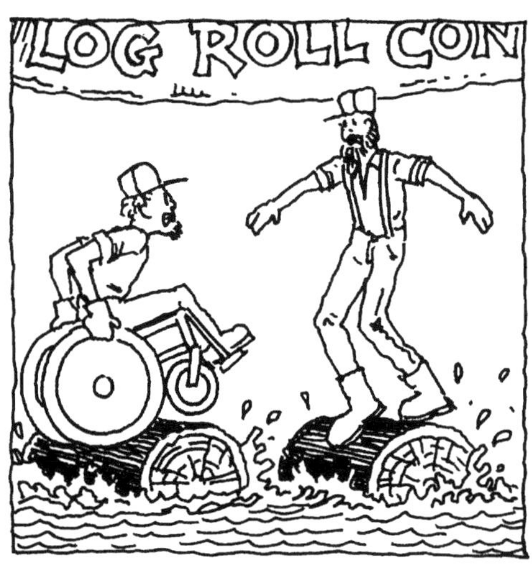

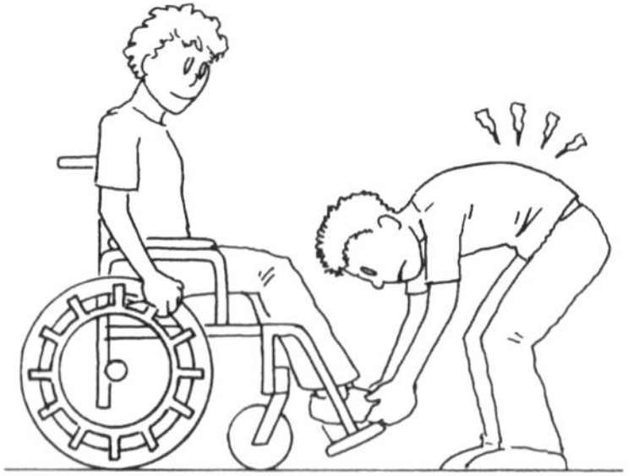

Bending from the waist can injure your back. Bend at the knees instead.

- Keep breathing. Holding your breath stiffens your muscles, making them easier to injure.
- When you get ready to lift, have the wheelchair user count to three. Lifting will be easier if everyone starts at the same time. If you start at different times, injuries may occur.

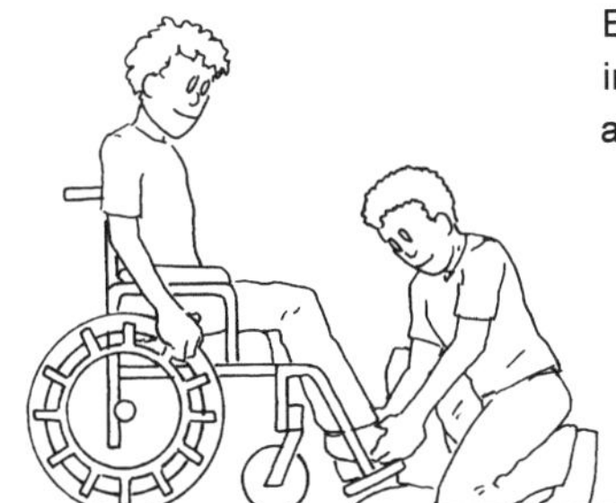

Bending at the knees and keeping your back upright can help you avoid injuring your back.

Using Safe Body Mechanics

Tipping their wheelchair into a wheelie

- Stand behind their wheelchair with your hands on the push handles or back posts, or use a spotting strap/sheet.
- Turn your body sideways and put your hip into the back of their wheelchair.
- Push down on the push handles or back posts, making sure to keep your back straight.
- Help balance their wheelchair in the wheelie position.

Assist up a curb

The wheelchair user should position his or her chair so the rear tires are backed against the curb. One assistant should be on the curb behind their wheelchair with hands on the push handles.

First assistant

- Grasp the push handles firmly. Stand with your legs apart from front to back.
- On the rider's count of three, lift and pull back on their wheelchair until it has rolled up onto the curb.
- Bend your back leg and shift your weight back onto it.
- Use your legs, not your back, to give you the strength you need to pull their wheelchair. Keep your back straight.

Second assistant

- Stand in front of the chair, facing the wheelchair user, with your toes approximately 12 inches from the chair.
- Lower yourself to the frame of their wheelchair by bending your knees. You should feel your hamstrings (the muscles on the backs of your thighs) working. Keep your back straight and do not lean forward.
- Grasp a structural portion of their wheelchair frame. Be prepared to lift and push from the front end of their wheelchair.
- On the rider's count of three, lift the front end of the wheelchair and push forward until all four wheels are safely on the curb. Use your legs for strength and keep your back straight. You should feel your quadriceps muscles (located above your knee and up your thigh) working.
- Stand up while keeping your back straight. You should feel your quadriceps muscles working.

Descending a curb facing backward

Stand behind their wheelchair with your hands on the push handles.

As the wheelchair user is backing off the curb, lean forward into the back of their wheelchair to help control the descent. Don't push so hard that you prevent their wheelchair from moving backward.

Use your legs for strength and keep your back straight.

Pushing up a ramp

Stand behind the wheelchair user with your hands on their wheelchair's push handles. Bend your knees and push off with your legs.

Keep your back straight as you push and use your legs for strength. Be sure you are not rounding your shoulders.

Pulling a wheelchair through snow or sand

Whenever possible, push instead of pull. Pushing is safer for your body. If you do need to pull, try to avoid pulling a wheelchair alone. It is best to have one person in front lifting the caster wheels while pulling forward, and another person pushing from behind.

First assistant

- Use a rope or a spotter strap and attach it to a structural portion on the front of the users wheelchair.
- Reach back and grasp the rope, keeping your elbows bent.
- As you move forward, lift up on the rope to unweight the casters and pull.
- Be sure to keep your back straight and use your legs for strength.

Second assistant

- Stand behind their wheelchair.
- Push down and forward on the push handles. This will help lift the caster wheels and provide forward momentum to their wheelchair.
- Bend your knees and push off with your legs.
- Keep your back straight as you push. Lean into the back of their wheelchair so you can use your legs, not your back, for strength. Be sure that your back is straight, not hunched, and you are not rounding your shoulders.

Section 5.2

Setting Limits and Offering Help

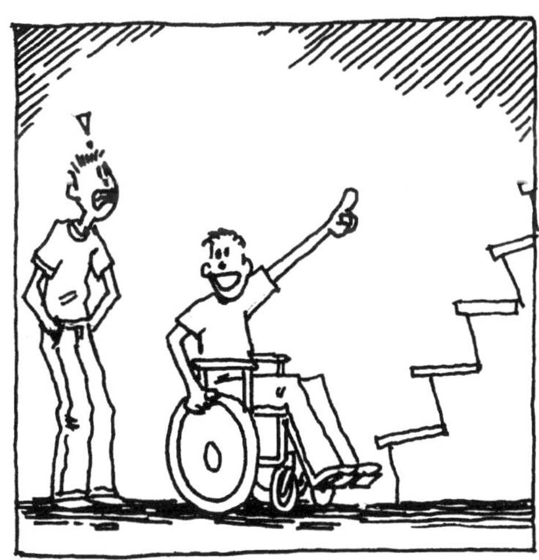

It can be hard to admit you have reached your limits. However, you should safeguard your own health and well-being. You need to know your limits and how to say "no" when you have reached them.

How to Say "No"

It is important to understand that you do not have to assist a wheelchair user if it will make you uncomfortable. This could result in injury to the wheelchair user or yourself. For example, pushing a wheelchair up a curb with an injured back could be painful and may cause further injury. Do not be afraid to say "No." The following are several ways to decline help:

- Politely decline by saying, "I don't feel comfortable or safe assisting you in that way." Explaining why you declined is often appreciated. However, if your reasons are personal, you have no obligation to explain yourself.
- Offer to find someone who can help. "I'm not able to assist you up this curb because I have a shoulder injury. Would you like me to find someone else?"
- Offer an alternative skill. "I'm not comfortable lifting your caster wheels onto the curb because I don't think I can lift the weight of your wheelchair. Can we try climbing it backward, and I'll pull from the push handles?"
- Offer an alternative route. "I'm concerned about trying to go down this steep hill. I don't think it's safe. The hill isn't as steep a little farther down the road."

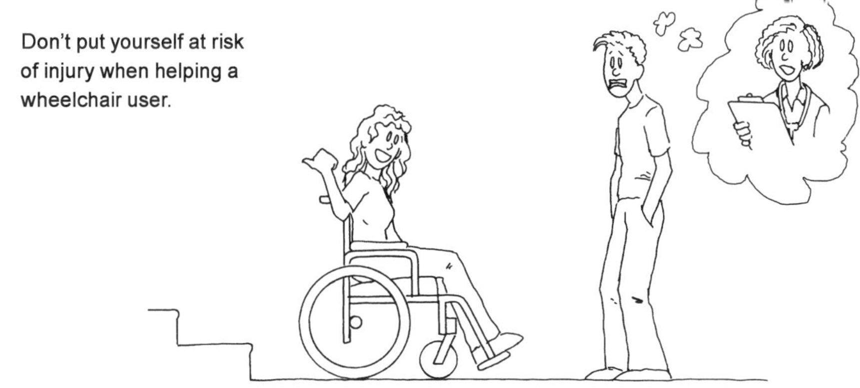

Don't put yourself at risk of injury when helping a wheelchair user.

Sometimes the wheelchair user will be surprised or become angry at your refusal to help even if you explained it. That's OK, you still need to protect yourself from injury.

Offering Assistance

Sometimes, watching a person who looks like he or she is struggling to complete a task is difficult. Keep in mind that the person may not want assistance; it may be important for him or her to accomplish the activity independently. It might be easier for the wheelchair user to do the activity alone than to explain to others how they can help. The wheelchair user might have had bad experiences in the past when people tried to help. The wheelchair user might even be out exercising. It may be difficult to watch, but you do not necessarily need to help the person. Don't be offended if the wheelchair user refuses your offer to help.

Only assist a wheelchair user when you are asked and/or have been given permission. If you think a wheelchair user might need assistance, offer. The wheelchair user may be in a position that looks precarious, but have the situation under control. Unexpected assistance might throw him or her off balance.

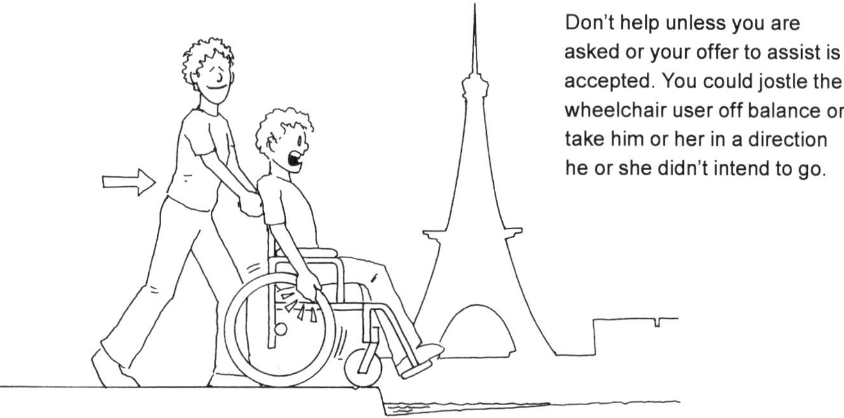

Don't help unless you are asked or your offer to assist is accepted. You could jostle the wheelchair user off balance or take him or her in a direction he or she didn't intend to go.

- Ask if the wheelchair user wants help. Avoid assertive statements such as, "Let me do this for you," which make it difficult for the wheelchair user to decline your help.
- Try wording your offer more casually. "Could you use a hand?" or "Can I help you out?"

If your offer to assist has been accepted, the wheelchair user is in charge. Ask the rider how you can help and follow his or her instructions. Ask the rider to talk you through the sequence before trying it, then work together to do it correctly.

- Do not push, lift, or pull unless the wheelchair user asks. Often you will be working together (e.g., to climb a curb, you may be pushing on the push handles as the wheelchair user pushes).
- Speak up if you feel in danger of injuring yourself by following the rider's instructions.
- Push or pull an occupied wheelchair only when the rider is actually pushing or pulling on the handrims. If you move the wheelchair when the rider is not expecting it or not holding on, you could cause the rider to fall out of the wheelchair.

Appendix A

The Americans with Disabilities Act of 1990

The Americans with Disabilities Act (ADA) was adopted as law in 1990 to ensure equal access to all individuals without regard to needs related to disability. This comprehensive law focuses on a number of areas, including accessibility to and within public buildings and services. The newest accessibility guidelines were published September 15, 2010 and became fully effective March 15, 2012. If you encounter problems with a building's accessibility, you should first speak with the building owner or manager and explain your problem. They may have been unaware of any accessibility difficulties, and could make immediate changes for you. If the building manager or owner is unwilling to help, the next step is to get other people in the building to talk to the management. Local advocacy groups, such as Centers for Independent Living, may offer intermediary services or provide alternative resources for addressing problems. If you cannot achieve a resolution of the problem using these methods, you can file a complaint with the Department of Justice. For information about filing a complaint, call the ADA information line at 800-514-0301. You can find more information about the ADA at www.ada.gov. You can find more information about Centers for Independent Living at the National Council for Independent Living website, www.ncil.org. You can also find the Center for Independent Living nearest you at this website.

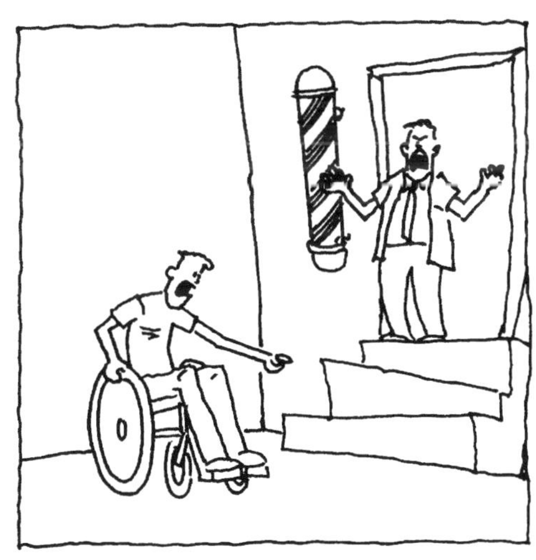

A problem might be as simple as a plant that was placed in front of the elevator buttons or within the clear passage of a hallway. It may be as complex as a multi-level building not serviced by an elevator or doorways that are too narrow for you to pass through.

Access Board

The U.S. Architectural and Transportation Barriers Compliance Board (Access Board) provides technical assistance on the ADA Accessibility Guidelines. The Access Board can be reached via the following:

- Voice: 800-872-2253
- TTY: 800-993-2822
- Internet address: www.access-board.gov

U.S. Department of Transportation

The ADA also addresses accessibility to transportation services. The United States Department of Transportation oversees this aspect of the ADA.

They can be reached via the following:

- Voice: 202-366-4000
- TTY: 800-877-8339
- Internet Address: www.dot.gov/accessibility

General ADA Information

You can reach the ADA Information Line to obtain ADA documents, ask questions, and obtain referrals via the following:

- Voice: 800-514-0301
- TTY: 800-514-0383
- Internet address: www.ada.gov

Appendix B

Accessories

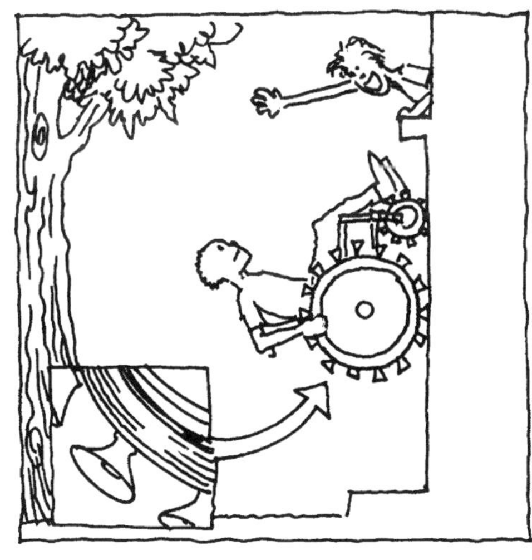

The availability of accessories for wheelchair users has expanded tremendously over the past few years. You could never need or use all the accessories available on the market- if you did, your chair would be bristling with enough gadgets and gizmos to rival a one-man novelty band. The accessories you choose will reflect your personal abilities, activities, skill level, and plain old personal preference. An accessory you use all the time might be merely a hindrance to another person. You will grow out of some accessories you found indispensable when you first started using a wheelchair. You may grow into other accessories as you gain experience with your chair. Below is a list of accessories, including a description, other common terms for the accessory, and the positives and negatives of using it.

airplane wheels – When quick release rear tires are removed, the wheelchair can roll on these wheels down an airplane aisle (these are slightly larger wheels than the little rollers on the anti-tippers).

Plus: allows you to pull yourself through a narrow door or down an airplane aisle

arm support panels – These plastic or metal guards attach to the arm supports, between the wheel and the rider.

Plus: keeps tire dirt on the outside of arm supports and away from your clothes

Minus: may reduce the effective width of your wheelchair seat; be sure to check the pressure on both sides of your hip bones

backpack – Bag designed to be worn on the back, it can also be attached to the back of a wheelchair by hooking the straps over the push handles or frame. Backpacks specifically designed for wheelchairs are also available.

Plus: can carry an assortment of supplies

Minus: additional weight on the back of the chair can increase likelihood of tipping over backward (if you plan to use a backpack often, practice skills with it on your chair)

bicycle lights – Lights designed to clip onto bicycles can increase your visibility to motorists. A white halogen lamp can act as a headlight. Blinking red lights can be clipped to the rear of your wheelchair to improve your visibility.

Plus: helps you view upcoming terrain; increases your visibility to motorists when traveling in the street; removable

Minus: require batteries; may not be as easy to mount on a wheelchair as to a bike

bike trailer – A wheeled cart that can be attached to the back of the wheelchair for added storage.

Plus: adds storage space if you need to transport a lot of things

Minus: limits maneuverability; requires more energy to propel wheelchair

caster wheel pins (caster wheel locks) – These pins lock the caster wheel in the forward or rearward trailing position.

Plus: stabilizes wheelchair when doing transfers; helpful when in rehab or to those new to using a wheelchair

Minus: usually unnecessary for more experienced wheelchair users

cellular phone

Plus: can be used to contact help in an emergency

Minus: must keep batteries charged; adds weight; additional expense to maintain; could create a distraction while maneuvering

chair guards (frame guards) – Chair guards are plastic or leather covers that fit over your wheelchair when you are not using it.

Plus: protects paint from damage caused by impact

Minus: You may need help to put it in place Unless you travel with it, it may not be where you need it

chest strap – A strap attached to the back of the wheelchair that crosses under your arms and over your chest. It can help prevent you from falling forward. Always use a lap belt if you are using a chest belt.

Plus: can prevent injury that might occur when falling forward out of wheelchair during sudden stops; provides additional trunk stability

Minus: locks you into your wheelchair, which may cause an injury if wheelchair falls over; can restrict mobility of trunk and/or buttocks

clothing guards (mud guards) – Plastic or nylon guards that stay between your wheels and clothes to keep you clean.

Plus: keeps clothing from getting soiled by dirt kicked up from tires

Minus: some people find clothing guards unsightly; may narrow the width of the seat

duct tape – Wide plastic tape embedded with fiber webbing for strength

Plus: very strong and sticky; can be used for temporary repairs while on the road

Minus: should not be used in place of proper wheelchair parts (e.g., not equivalent to a bolt); may leave a sticky residue after removal

running brakes – Used to slow a moving wheelchair. Rare, but available on some European-made wheelchairs, also as an aftermarket product, you can add to your wheels if needed.

Plus: may be helpful when moving on downward slopes

Minus: adds weight to the wheelchair; may interfere with usual propulsion and rear wheel removal

electrical tape – Thin, stretchy plastic tape that is used to bind electrical wires. Comes in many colors.

Plus: can be used for on the road repairs until you can get home and fix the problem properly

Minus: not as sticky or strong as duct tape

flags – A tall, flexible rod with a triangular flag (usually vinyl or plastic); usually comes in a fluorescent color. Mounts to the back of your wheelchair to improve your visibility.

Plus: helps prevent accidents by making you more visible to motorists

Minus: many dislike the way the flag looks, can get caught on low-hanging obstacles

flashlight - Useful when traveling along dark streets and to improve your visibility to others. For easy access, use a Velcro™ strap to attach it to the frame of your wheelchair.

Plus: can be used to look for lost objects and to help perform emergency repairs

Minus: people with limited hand function may have difficulty operating

fold-down briefcase rest (luggage carrier) – Small lever that attaches to each foot support side rails. When raised, can hold a briefcase or travel bag at your feet, where you can access it easily. Folds down and out of the way when not in use.

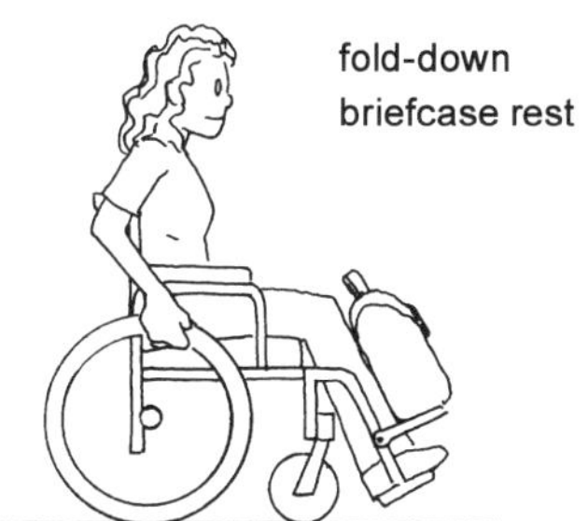

Plus: keeps items conveniently located within easy reach; folds up when not in use

Minus: heavy bag may tip wheelchair in the forward direction

foot straps – Straps that attach to the foot supports and loop over the top of each foot to keep them from sliding forward off the foot supports.

Plus: prevent feet from falling forward off foot supports; limit the chance of injury or accident caused by feet hitting the ground in front of the foot supports; will prevent legs from falling onto face in a backward fall

Minus: need to be released for transfers; if you fall from your wheelchair, your feet will stay attached to the foot supports and this can be dangerous

gloves – Gloves with grips such as plastic strips or dots on the palms.

Plus: keep your hands clean; helps prevent blisters; helps prevent hands from sliding on the handrims; can protect hands from friction burns when braking down a steep grade

Minus: can be hot to wear; wear out quickly

hand bike – bicycle that can be pedaled with the hands and arms.

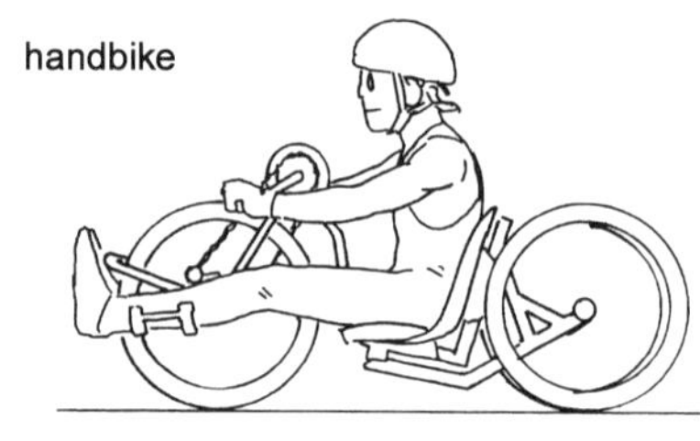

handiwipes (wet naps, baby-wipes) – Wet cloths used for cleaning hands and face. Available in plastic dispensers or in individual packets.

Plus: can clean your hands when a sink is not nearby or accessible

Minus: occupy limited carrying space

head rests – Mounts to the back of the wheelchair and used to support the head, as in car seats.

Plus: reduce chance of whiplash if head is snapped back in an auto accident

Minus: may limit sight when looking behind

hill climbers (grade aids) – Hill climbers attach to the wheelchair on or near the parking brake. When engaged, they allow the wheelchair to roll forward, but prevent it from rolling backward.

Plus: reduces the likelihood of rolling backward on an incline

Minus: may interfere with usual wheelchair propulsion

key clasps – Small clasps with key rings attached that can hook keys to the frame of your wheelchair.

Plus: easy access to keys; keeps keys visible to limit theft from a backpack

Minus: the clasp may be hard to open for persons with limited mobility in their hands

lap belt – A belt worn across the lap to prevent forward falls out of the wheelchair. A lap belt should always be used with a chest support. Belt clasps come in many different styles.

Plus: can prevent injury that might occur when falling forward out of wheelchair, due to a sudden stop; provides stability to allow independent function

Minus: locks you into your wheelchair, which may cause an injury if wheelchair tips completely forward; can restrict mobility of trunk and/or buttocks

leg straps – Straps that hold the legs to the wheelchair frame just above the foot supports.

Plus: prevent feet from falling off foot supports, limiting chance of injury caused by feet getting stuck behind foot supports; useful on rough terrain; will prevent legs from flopping onto the face in a backward fall

Minus: may interfere with swing-away foot supports

mirrors - Mirrors mounted onto the frame of your wheelchair can be used similarly to mirrors on a car.

Plus: helps you see what's behind you

Minus: will not help you see motorists, pedestrians, and bicyclists in your blind spot (the area just to the side and behind you that is not reflected in the mirror)

noise maker – A horn or bell attached to your wheelchair can be used to signal motorists, pedestrians, and bicyclists. Can be purchased at bicycle shops.

Plus: notifies motorists, pedestrians, and bicyclists of your presence to reduce the possibility of collision

Minus: some do not like the way horns look or sound; may be difficult to reach and activate

patch kit – A patch kit will help fix flat tires. You will still need a pump to fill the patched tire with air.

Plus: permits you to repair tire punctures on the road

Minus: adds weight to your supplies

pump – Can be used to inflate tires that need air.

Plus: helps you avoid being stranded

Minus: adds weight

reflective tape – Brightly colored plastic or vinyl tape that reflects light aimed at it; can be attached to your wheelchair and/or clothing.

Plus: makes you more visible to motorists

Minus: may appear unsightly to some wheelchair users

reflectors – Plastic disks or rectangles that reflect light aimed at them; can be attached to the spokes, frame, or back of a wheelchair to improve your visibility to motorists. Recommended if wheeling in the roadway where vehicular traffic is anticipated.

seat pouch – Cloth pouches specifically designed to be attached under wheelchair seats. A fanny pack (nylon or cloth pouches worn around the waist) can be modified to serve as a seat pouch.

Plus: provides additional storage space; under-seat position provides better security than a backpack

Minus: people with little or no upper-body strength may have difficulty reaching under-seat pouches

shoulder harness – Strap that fits over your shoulders and hooks around the back of a wheelchair to help keep you upright and bolster your forward stability.

Plus: can prevent injury that might occur when falling forward out of wheelchair due to sudden stops

Minus: locks you into your wheelchair which may cause an injury if it tips completely forward; may limit reach even more than a chest strap

spoke guards – Plastic disks that fit over your outer spokes; function as a hubcap for the rear wheels.

Plus: protects spokes from being damaged, protects fingers from getting caught in spokes, useful in sporting events where wheelchairs tend to collide

Minus: add weight; can degrade quickly

supports (postural support devices, trunk supports) – Padding that can be added to a wheelchair seat and/or back to improve the seating position of the rider. May include chest straps, lap belts, side-to-side supports, and hip guides.

Plus: provides stability to allow independent function

Minus: may restrict mobility of trunk and/or buttocks; may interfere with transfers

Swiss Army Knife (multi-purpose tool) – Can function as an all-in-one tool kit; depending on the model, it can include screwdrivers, scissors, knife blades, files, pliers, and tweezers.

Plus: handy while out and about, saves time spent looking for tools

Minus: requires good hand function to operate

tray (lap tray) – A flat removable surface (usually plastic) that mounts to the frame and extends over your lap. It can be used as a surface for eating, playing games, reading, writing, etc.

Plus: can provide a good substitute for tables when available tables and counters are too low to wheel under

Minus: adds weight; may feel and look awkward; limits ability to access other surfaces

web cradle – A square piece of mesh that attaches below the seat and is used for storage.

Plus: additional storage for books, clothes, etc.

Minus: stored items may get dirty

Appendix C

References and Resources

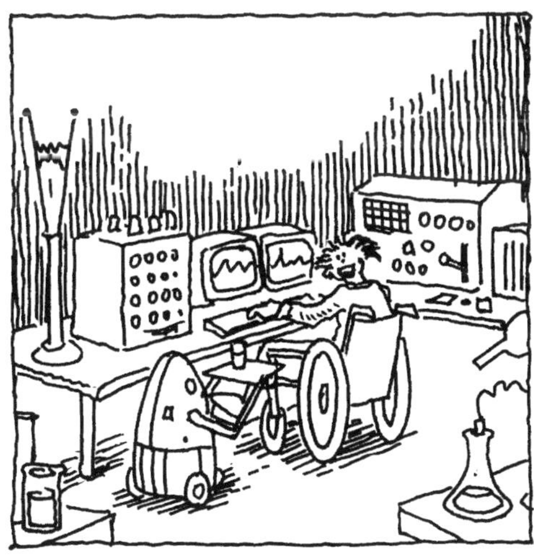

If you are interested in obtaining additional information about wheelchairs and mobility skills, there are a number of resources you can tap into with a visit, a phone call, a letter, or an internet connection.

Centers for Independent Living (CIL)

Most communities have a Center for Independent Living (also called Independent Living Centers, or ILCs). These are run by and for people with disabilities. Their mission is to help people with disabilities live more independently and as productive and fully participating members of society. You can find more information about Centers for Independent Living at the National Council on Independent Living website at www.ncil.org.

Rehabilitation Centers

The rehabilitation center in your area may have facilities you can use to try out equipment and see which devices might benefit you. They may recommend an evaluation by either an occupational or physical therapist, a RESNA-certified assistive technology professional (ATP), or seating and mobility specialist (SMS). These professionals can often provide you with insight into your abilities and potential needs and may be able to direct you toward other helpful accessories. Your rehabilitation center may also refer you to other centers that can better meet your specific needs.

Medical Equipment Suppliers

Medical equipment suppliers represent equipment manufacturers and should be able to help you make choices compatible with your lifestyle. Remember that these companies are in the business of selling equipment, so you need to be an educated consumer and look further than the salesperson. The National registry of rehabilitation technology suppliers (NRRTS) has a registry of equipment suppliers. You can find more information at www.nrrts.org.

When buying equipment, consider the resources and reliability of the supplier. Ask them about their repair policies. For instance, will they loan you equipment when yours is being repaired? Are they helpful on the telephone? Do they seem willing to spend time telling you about the pros and cons of the variety of equipment? Will they help you adjust and re-adjust your equipment? The supplier might be willing to give you the names of a few of their customers . Contact these people to determine how they feel about the supplier's services.

Equipment Manufacturers

Most wheelchair and related equipment manufacturers have websites and toll-free numbers to assist you in gathering information. They will often refer you to a local supplier or others in your area who are familiar with their products. Some manufacturers have technical assistance departments that may be able to help you with specific questions about modifications, adjustments, or repairs. Some manufacturers publish documents in addition to their wheelchair owner's manuals. You can talk with your local supplier about getting documents from any of the manufacturers. The following publications, provided by Invacare, Corp., were used as references in this manual:

Educational Series–Volume 5: *The Wheelchair user.*
Invacare Corporation, 899 Cleveland St., Elyria, OH 44036.

Educational Series–Volume 6: *Maintenance & Adjustments for Wheelchairs.*
Invacare Corporation, 899 Cleveland St., Elyria, OH 44036.

Educational Series–Volume 7: *Safety/Handling of Wheelchairs.*
Invacare Corporation, 899 Cleveland St., Elyria, OH 44036.

Other Wheelchair Users

Find people in your community who have similar interests and needs. Other people often have recommendations for equipment and you can combine their information with the recommendations you get from rehab professionals and equipment suppliers. By learning as much as you can, you will be able to make more informed decisions about your equipment.

Professional Organizations

Some professional organizations may be able to provide you with information directly or refer you to members in your area who may be familiar with similar circumstances to yours. Six such organizations are included here:

American Physical Therapy Association (APTA)
1111 N. Fairfax St.
Alexandria, VA 22314
(703) 684-2782 voice, (703) 684-7343 fax
www.apta.org

American Occupational Therapy Association (AOTA)
4720 Montgomery Lane, Suite 200
Bethesda, MD 20814-3449
(301) 652-2682 voice, (301) 652-7711 fax
www.aota.org

Disabled Sports USA (DSUSA)
451 Hungerford Drive, Suite 100
Rockville, MD 20850
(301) 217-0960 voice
www.dsusa.org

National Registry of Rehabilitation Technology Suppliers (NRRTS)
112 E. 6th Street
P.O. Box 1091
Walsenburg, CO 81089
(719) 738-5770 voice, (888) 480-7522 fax
www.nrrts.org

Paralyzed Veterans of America Spinal Cord Injury Education Foundation
801 18th Street NW
Washington, DC 20006-3517
(202) 416-7652 voice, (202) 416-7641 fax
www.pvaresearch.org

Rehabilitation Engineering and Assistive Technology Society of North America (RESNA)
1700 N. Moore St., Suite 1540
Arlington, VA 22209
(703) 524-6686 voice, (703) 524-6630
www.resna.org

Publications

Active Living Magazine
www.disabilitytodaynetwork.com

Journal of Rehabilitation Research & Development (JRRD)
103 South Gay Street
Baltimore, MD 21202-4061
www.rehab.research.va.gov/jrrd/

Magazine of the American Association of People with Disabilities (AAPD)
2013 H Street, NW, 5th Floor
Washington, DC 20006
(202) 457-0046 voice, (866) 536-4461 fax
www.aapd.com

New Mobility
United Spinal Association
75-20 Astoria Boulevard
East Elmhurst, NY 11370
(800) 404 2898
www.newmobility.com

Paraplegia News
Paralyzed Veterans of America
2111 East Highland Avenue, Suite 180
Phoenix, AZ 85016-4702
(602) 224-0500 voice, (602) 224-0507 fax
http://pvamag.com/pn/

Sports 'n Spokes
This magazine publishes annual articles comparing available wheelchair models.
Paralyzed Veterans of America
2111 East Highland Avenue, Suite 180
Phoenix, AZ 85016-4702
(602) 224-0500 voice, (602) 224-0507 fax
http://pvamag.com/sns/

Appendix D

Wheelchair Skills Program (WSP)©

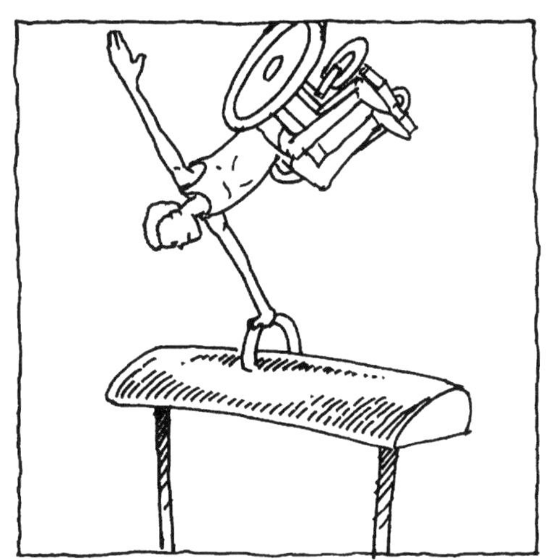

We are including the Wheelchair Skills Test (WST)© for your personal use. There is a manual with instructions for each step of this form. This manual and related materials can be downloaded from:

www.wheelchairskillsprogram.ca/eng/testers.php

For further information, contact: wsp@dal.ca

There are many more resources at http://www.wheelchairskillsprogram.ca/

Warnings

The wheelchair skills described and illustrated in the WSP can be dangerous and result in severe injury if attempted without the assistance of trained personnel. Wheelchair skills are potentially dangerous, some more so than others. Attempting these skills may not be appropriate for some wheelchair users or caregivers. If the skills are attempted, for assessment or training purposes, an experienced spotter should be available to intervene.

Acknowledgements

This work would not have been possible without the excellent papers, textbooks and training manuals that have been published by others. This literature is too extensive to cite here, but has been more specifically acknowledged in the reference sections of our papers published about the WSP (see web site).

The WSP was developed for clinical and research purposes. We thank the many people who have provided advice and assistance in the development of the WSP. Funding support has been received from a number of local, regional and national funding agencies. We have avoided naming individual colleagues and funding agencies in this document because the list is constantly growing. However, the names of these people and agencies are noted in specific published papers, listed elsewhere.

Wheelchair Skills Test (WST) Version 4.2 Form
Manual Wheelchairs Operated by Their Users

Name of wheelchair user: ______________________

Tester: ______________________ Date: ______________

#	Individual Skill	Capacity Score* (0-2)	Trainging Goal? (Y/N)	Comments
1	Rolls forwards (10 m)			
2	Rolls backwards (2 m)			
3	Turns while moving forwards (90°)			
4	Turns while moving backwards (90°)			
5	Turns in place (180°)			
6	Maneuvers sideways (0.5 m)			
7	Gets through hinged door			
8	Reaches high object (1.5 m)			
9	Picks object up from floor			
10	Relieves weight from buttocks (3 sec)			
11	Transfers to and from bench			
12	Folds and unfolds wheelchair			
13	Rolls 100 m			
14	Avoids moving obstacles			
15	Ascends 5° incline			
16	Descends 5° incline			
17	Ascends 10° incline			
18	Descends 10° incline			
19	Rolls across side-slope (5°)			
20	Rolls on soft surface (2 m)			
21	Gets over gap (15 cm)			
22	Gets over threshold (2 cm)			
23	Ascends low curb (5 cm)			
24	Descends low curb (5 cm)			
25	Ascends curb (15 cm)			
26	Descends curb (15 cm)			
27	Performs stationary wheelie (30 sec)			
28	Turns in place in wheelie position (180°)			
29	Descends 10° incline in wheelie position			
30	Descends curb in wheelie position (15 cm)			
31	Gets from ground into wheelchair			
32	Descends stairs			
	Total score:*		%	

*See score options and formula for calculating total score on page 2

WST 4.2 Form for Manual Wheelchairs operated by Their Users
Originally approved for distribution and use: April 3, 2013; Current version: May 24, 2013 1

Comments:

Training goals:

Person (if any) and address to whom the test subject would like a copy of the report to be sent:

Scoring Options for Individual Skills

Score	Score	What this means
Pass	2	Task independently and safely accomplished without any difficulty.
Pass with difficulty	1	The evaluation criteria are met, but the subject experienced some difficulty worthy of note.
Fail	0	Task incomplete or unsafe.
Not possible	NP	The wheelchair does not have the parts to allow this skill.
Testing error	TE	Testing of the skill was not sufficiently well observed to provide a score.

Formula for Calculating Total Scores

Total Capacity Score = sum of individual capacity scores/([32 – # of NP and TE scores] x 2) X 100%

Copies can be downloaded from www.wheelchairskillsprogram.ca